Losing
My Mind

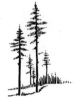

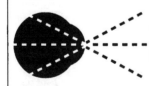

This Large Print Book carries the
Seal of Approval of N.A.V.H.

Losing
My Mind

An Intimate Look at
Life with Alzheimer's

Thomas DeBaggio

Thorndike Press • Waterville, Maine

Published in 2002 by arrangement with The Free Press, a division of Simon & Schuster, Inc.

Thorndike Press Large Print Senior Lifestyles Series.

The tree indicium is a trademark of Thorndike Press.

The text of this Large Print edition is unabridged. Other aspects of the book may vary from the original edition.

Set in 16 pt. Plantin by Liana M. Walker.

Printed in the United States on permanent paper.

Library of Congress Cataloging-in-Publication Data

DeBaggio, Thomas, 1942–
    Losing my mind : an intimate look at life with Alzheimer's / Thomas DeBaggio.
      p. cm.
    Previously published: New York : Free Press, c2002.
    ISBN 0-7862-4376-7 (lg. print : hc : alk. paper)
    1. DeBaggio, Thomas, 1942– — Health.   2. Alzheimer's disease — Patients — Virginia — Biography.   3. Large type books. I. Title.
RC523 .D43 2002
362.1′96831′0092—dc21
   [B]   2002020378

To my wife, Joyce,
may she always remember our good days.
And to my son, Francesco,
who made every day worth remembering.
And in memory of Connie and Carl who
made me,
and left too soon.
Thanks for the time of my life.

Acknowledgments

Many friends helped with this project, as they have in the past, and again I owe them much.

Joyce and Francesco spent many patient hours listening to me tell stories and share frustrations, and they helped guide me in this endeavor. Their story is hidden in the corners of almost every page of this book. Without their patience, help, and love this book could not have been written.

Tammy Boggs, Rick Tagg, Dottie Jacobsen, and Tina Zaras, wonderful friends, watched my battle and helped me in many varied ways, some unknown to them. Rob Lively, a friend of longstanding, lent more than moral support.

My sister, Mary Ann Lovett, opened her heart and helped me remember her role in my growing up, while my cousins Suzanne and John Cain called regularly from the West Coast to remind me of events when we were together in Eldora, and to cheer me. My longtime friend Rob Hurwitt made suggestions on the finished manuscript and helped reduce typos.

Pete Dawson, our family's ribald historian, traced evidence of Alzheimer's in the DeBiaggio family and provided levity. His family chronicle of the Dapalonia and DeBiaggio families provided some useful background that was outside my memory.

My good friends Susan Belsinger in Maryland and Carolyn Dille in California kept my spirits high with frequent telephone calls.

Linda Ligon of Interweave Press, a friend of many years, encouraged my writing over the years, often in the best way, with money for work published in her magazines and books, and she prodded me to keep going during these tough times.

Noah Adams was helpful in many ways.

I am indebted to Dr. Colleen Blanchfield, a neurologist with a large heart for her patients and a sensitivity for their humanity. She is an honor to her profession.

I am particularly indebted to Jonathan Lazear and Christi Cardenas for their help and their enthusiasm for my writing.

My profound thanks to those men and women, and mice, around the world who work to understand Alzheimer's and bring its awful nightmares to an end.

Author's Note

This is a book balanced between the wonder of childhood and the tottering age of memory. I used an unconventional multilayered style in this book to illustrate memory's many faults and strengths. It is an attempt to show the parameters of long- and short-term memory and how Alzheimer's works to destroy the present and the past. To do this I set up three narrative lines.

In my notes, I call the first narrative the Baby Book. It deals with long-term memory from my first awareness through the early 1970s.

A second narrative intersects the first, relating stories of humiliation and loss. It contains rough details of my tangle with Alzheimer's. This narrative represents a mind-clogged, uncertain present. It is filled with memory lapses and language difficulties and the sudden barks of disappointment and loss.

A third stream is filled with recent Alzheimer's research. All this is mixed together, as it is in the brain, and follows a pattern of its own.

Memory is hunger.

— Ernest Hemingway in *A Moveable Feast*

*I am going to tell the story of my life
in an alphabet of ashes.*

— Blas De Otero in *Twenty Poems*

That January, my fifty-seventh birthday, was pleasant and eventful and I began to adjust to middle age. I no longer noticed how small facial lines became wrinkles. I was active and happy. My son Francesco, home from California, joined Joyce and me in the family herb-growing business in Virginia. I was equipped with a thin body free of aches and pains. I looked forward to a life to rival my Midwestern grandmother's 104 years. I was buoyant and displayed, occasionally, the unbecoming arrogance of youth.

Then came a beautiful spring day later that year. It was the day after the tests were finished and the results reviewed. It was the day I was diagnosed with Alzheimer's. What time had hidden was now revealed. Genetic secrets, locked inside before my birth, were now in the open. I became a new member in the parade of horror created by Alzheimer's.

At first I viewed the diagnosis as a death sentence. Tears welled up in my eyes uncontrollably; spasms of depression grabbed me by the throat. I was nearer to death than I anticipated. A few days later I realized good might come of this. After forty years of pussyfooting with words, I finally had a story of hell to tell.

. . . .

My parents grew up in an orderly, gentle time, or so they remembered it. Their epoch was also full of dirty secrets, enslavement, lynching, and two murderous convulsive world wars. It was a time to need luck. They escaped the influenza epidemic of 1918 and made it through the Great Depression of the thirties when food and jobs were scarce. Luck was with them in small Iowa towns named Eldora and Colfax.

Instead of focusing on the explosive reality of their time, they created a happier personal interval of their own imagining. This in turn created a great optimism in me and a gentle narrative of childhood tranquility. Soon I was scared and uplifted, as were they, by the time of my time, a world of conflagration, disorder, hope, ugliness, great beauty, and unnecessary death. Yet the imaginative world of kindness and promise they passed to me always remained untouched by the ugliness of congested cities, immoral wars, and encompassing greed.

Here I am at the moment of truth and all I

can muster are hot screams and scribbled graffiti torn from my soul. Moments of slithering memory now define my life.

After a short, mild winter, a vivid spring settled around us. The weather was tame and herbs filled a sunny patch next to the greenhouse. They were strong and vigorous now, especially the rosemaries, the thymes, the lavenders. Their scents perfumed the air when I brushed by them.

The sun warmed the earth steadily and it was possible to spade and plant a kitchen garden with early seed crops of succulent lettuce to sweeten and color our meals. It was a spring in which you could be happy and a little carefree. There was much the earth had to say and you could hear it if you stayed quiet and listened intently.

There was something else that spring and it was unnamable. As with all unknowns, it was unsettling and had nothing to do with the weather. It was not something that gentle rains, bright sunny days, and an optimistic outlook would cure. It was an anonymous presence, yet I could feel its uneasy cadence. My memory, which had been a sacred touchstone, was failing long before I expected. I was losing the ability to remember things important to me. I had difficulty recognizing the names of many of my plants, and even friends I saw infrequently. I was fifty-seven this year, and not eager to acknowledge that now I might be tied to a teetering mind that had begun a slow descent into silence.

A time or two I complained out loud that I could not remember things that the year before had been brightly colored and detailed. I brushed off those incidents as forgetfulness due to stress, and there was stress aplenty, as there had been always. Stress and worry were steady partners in my backyard farming, just as it was for the farmer in the great, flat Midwest with hundreds of acres of rich, black earth.

I made a living in my backyard for twenty-four years, growing and selling as many as 100,000 herb and vegetable plants from my greenhouse each spring. The entire operation, situated on a 5,000-square-foot lot, contained our family home and a 1,600-square-foot greenhouse. It marked me as a new breed of urban farmer who scorned grass and its wasteful, demanding cultivation. I made a living off the land by selling directly to gardeners the potted plants I started from seeds and rooted cuttings and grew carefully in the greenhouse.

It had always been tough outwitting nature. It was a struggle the mind and body accepted willingly by turning work into games. It was serious and enjoyable play for me, but it was also my livelihood. My family depended on my ability to tame nature and use my guileless skills to attract customers. From the beginning, my tangle with urban farming was a test of my strength and acumen against nature's unpredictability.

I was completing a doctor visit, a regimen that was new and uncertain to me, when my physician asked, "Is there anything you want to tell me?" He is a thoughtful, no-nonsense man with a sly sense of humor, and the question may have been the kind of thing he often says as he winds up a session with a patient.

"Yes, there is," I said. He said nothing and waited for my words. "I am having trouble remembering things that are basic to my work, things I have known and now can't remember."

There was silence while he looked at me. "I can give you a referral," he said quickly, careful not to confuse or cheapen my predicament with some offhand remark. "And I will have the nurse take additional blood samples for the doctor I am sending you to."

I made an appointment to have the blood drawn the next day at the clinic. After I dressed, one of the doctor's assistants gave me a piece of paper with another physician's name, address, and telephone number. I had never seen the name before and it meant nothing to me, but the address was a prestigious university hospital. The first four of many vials of blood yet to be drawn were taken the next day.

. . . .

*Alzheimer's disease was named nearly 100 years ago for Alois Alzheimer, a German who first described the grisly effects of the disease. To gather his knowledge, he cut away the tops of several skulls from people who died of a mind-destroying malady, leaving them helpless, speechless, and as useless as a year-old carrot. He was probably the first to see inside a diseased brain and view the signature features of Alzheimer's, the sticky amyloid plaques and the twisted, hair-like threads of the neurofibrillary tangles.*Alzheimer's method of diagnosis after death remains the only way to be absolutely certain of the disease even today. As a result, questions often remain about a diagnosis, a condition that eager charlatans use to their advantage.

In a test of my memory and ability to learn new things, I came out "severely impaired" according to my neuropsychological evaluation. Doctors say I am at the beginning of the disease's onslaught.

For a guy hardly sick in his life, this is a large, corrosive event. I am not alone. In a few years nearly half of those who reach eighty years old will have the disease, according to the Alzheimer's Association. I am not so lucky in another way. The disease is known to strike as early as thirty, but only a tiny minority falls in its clutches before the mid-sixties. At fifty-seven the disease has been active in me for longer than I know.

Instead of bringing this disease into sunshine where we can learn about it and do something, it has been too often hidden and misunderstood, closeted to protect the living from its frightening consequences. Alzheimer's does not have the drama of a heart attack or the thud of an automobile wreck.

Our understanding of the disease has been, until recently, held hostage by lack of knowledge. Now we know it was not undefined evil, profligate activity, or witchcraft causing the strange behavior created by the disease. We are close to understanding mechanisms triggering this ghostly malady. The disease, or its potential, appears to rest secretly inside us until its evil time arises and a languid torture begins. This is a disease probably not caused by something you did to your body. It is, most likely, a consequence of bad luck, subtle effects activated in the brain, and parents who carried corrupted genes.

The disease works slowly, destroying the mind, stealing life in a tedious, silent dance of death. Slowly the memory is impaired, and then you wander in a world without certainty and names. Yesterdays disappear, except those long ago. Eventually there is a descent into silence and a dependence on caretakers. Hands other than yours feed and bathe you. A cipher takes your place amid the tubes and tragedy. By the end, Alzheimer's leaves its victims silent, quivering in their flesh, awaiting the last rites. Some common illness often takes credit on the death certificate.

I am alone and I can hear water running somewhere in the house. I don't remember going to the bathroom. Who else turned on the water?

This is an unfinished story of a man dying

in slow motion. It is filled with graffiti, sorrow, frustration, and short bursts of anger. While the narrator suffers his internal spears, he tries to surround himself with memories in a wan attempt to make sense of his life and give meaning to its shallow substance before he expires. Although incomplete, the story is full of sadness and missed opportunity, a lonely tale of the human condition. Behind it is hope, the tortured luck of a last chance.

My Midwestern mother and father conducted a torrid romance, according to cousin Pete. Every time my father returned to college after a holiday in Eldora, he sought a confessional priest, Pete remembers.

The secret transformation of my mother into a Catholic must have shocked my Lutheran grandmother, but she remained loyal to her daughter. My father became a lawyer, my mother a teacher.

Books set imaginations on fire in earlier times, and they continue to inspire and inform, but television and movies replaced much of the storytelling for my generation and left us hungry and naked, shivering for substance.

Alzheimer's disease is an irreversible, progressive brain disorder that occurs gradually and results in memory loss, unusual behavior, personality changes, and a decline in thinking abilities. These losses are related to the death of brain cells and the breakdown of the connections between them. The course of the disease varies from person to person, as does the rate of decline. On average, Alzheimer's patients live for 8 to 10 years after they are diagnosed; however, the disease can last for up to 20 years.

— "PROGRESS REPORT
ON ALZHEIMER'S DISEASE,"
NATIONAL INSTITUTE ON AGING, 1999

This may be my last chance to dream.

The inspiration for this book appeared a few days after I was diagnosed with Alzheimer's. It was to be a word picture of the outside and inside, present and past, of a man's naked struggle with the unknown on his way to trembling silence and unexplainable torment without the torturer. It was a story of unleashed anger and beauty brought forth by an unseen illness, incurable and relatively long-term in duration. I knew I was unable to write about all stages of Alzheimer's because the disease causes cognitive decline and I will lapse into a world without language and memory.

With any untreatable, disabling malady, victims become sensitized to every movement of their body, every breath, searching for change and studying the course of the illness until it threatens to destroy friendships and the love of those around them. Writing about it may be a way to legitimize my almost continuous contemplation of the subject, and I hope it will allow me to leave thoughts of the disease locked up in the computer while I conduct everyday affairs.

It is my intention to stay in the open with no secrets. I will hide nothing, not even the inevitable self-absorption typical of such a disease. To retreat from my lonely internal immersion with myself and the disease, I started a diary that has become this book, as unique perhaps as the disease itself.

Sweet memory, the unreliable handmaiden of the past.

I was born in a wicked midwinter Iowa

snowstorm and my father, proud and happy after the delivery, took the news to his parents in their little restaurant a few steps from the hospital in Eldora, Iowa. I was taken home to a small white house where many of my parents' friends arrived with good wishes and grand hopes for the future.

———

Much news was made of the possible link between aluminum and Alzheimer's when larger than expected amounts of the metal were discovered in the brains of some people who died of Alzheimer's. Worried that aluminum might somehow promote the disease, many people began to throw away cans, cookware, cosmetics, antacids, deodorants, and other items containing the metal. However, studies of people exposed to large quantities of aluminum revealed no increased incidence of dementia. Most likely, the deposition of aluminum in brain tissue is a result — not a cause — of the factors that underlie the dementia. (Incidentally, more aluminum leaches into soft drinks from glass bottles than from aluminum cans, which are coated with a fine veneer of plastic.)
— THE JOHNS HOPKINS WHITE PAPERS, "MEMORY," 1999

I am back from the drugstore with my packet of pills, prescription number 736631 from the CVS pharmacy, four blocks up the street. The pills have in them a pharmaceutical called Aricept, the trade name for donepezil HCl, the commonly prescribed medication for Alzheimer's at the time. The doctor told me the most common side effect is diarrhea. Boy, was he right.

I don't know whether to love these little round things or hate them. The pills are tiny and buff colored and on one side a "10" is stamped into it to designate it as a 10-milligram tablet and on the opposite side is the word Aricept. I started taking half of one of the tablets at bedtime. After five days, I was directed to take an entire tablet when I go to bed (later I began taking a second tablet before breakfast). Aricept was the second pharmaceutical developed for Alzheimer's and is now the most widely used medicine available, but at its best it can slow the destruction of brain cells temporarily.

The doctor also prescribed two over-the-counter medications to take daily: two vitamin E soft gels, each 1,000 international units, about 6,666 times more than the normally recommended dose, and a single Ibuprofen tablet. This combination of drug and vitamins is all medical science can do for me nearly 100 years after Alzheimer's was scientifically described. It seems a weak armada to defend against eager memory destroyers working in my brain. I am a citizen of a country that has sent mankind to the moon. It is sadly ironic but that is all medical science can do, when we spend billions to send men into outer space to look at rocks.

I am happy today. I realized this was not yet a posthumous tale.

———

The brain does many things to ensure our survival. It integrates, regulates, initiates, and controls functions in the whole body, with the help of motor and sensory nerves outside of the brain and spinal cord. The brain governs thinking, personality, mood, and the senses. We can speak, move, and remember because of complex chemical processes that take place in our brains. The brain also regulates body functions that happen without our knowledge or directions, such as digestion of food.
— "PROGRESS REPORT
ON ALZHEIMER'S DISEASE,"
NATIONAL INSTITUTE ON AGING, 1999

★ ★ ★

How do you express the true nature of tears in words? How do you define the limits of evil born of a secret disease? These thoughts lie silently on my mind and work their way through my body.

In geriatric clinics, about 5 to 10 percent of the patients seen for memory impairment have reversible dementia due to medication. Some of the medications that may cause memory impairment include the anti-inflammation drug prednisone (Deltasone, Orasone, for example); heartburn drugs such as cimetidine (Tagamet), famotidine (Pepcid), and ranitidine (Zantac); anti-anxiety/sedative drugs such as triazolam (Halcion), alprazolam (Xanax), or diazapern (Valium); or even insulin, which at too high a dose can cause hypoglycemia (abnormally low blood sugar). . . . Alcohol is the most prevalent intoxicant implicated in dementia. Fortunately, as is often the case with other drugs, the negative effects of alcohol on intellectual abilities can be reversed with abstinence, though chronic abuse may lead to permanent damage.
— THE JOHNS HOPKINS WHITE PAPERS, "MEMORY," 1999

Before the end of my first year, my mother and father became immigrants and took up residence in an apartment in Washington, DC. It was a sleepy Southern town with a twang, and racial segregation was strictly enforced. Half a continent separated me and my birthplace, and more than miles divided them. My father went to work for the Bureau of Narcotics. It was half a lifetime, and many changes and surprises, before he returned to live in Eldora again.

I don't know if any of us can be prepared for what is to come. It is hard to prepare for the sly tricks and sorrows of tomorrow. Better we hug each other more often and forget the creeping sadness that we know will overcome us.

. . . .

The lovely long spring with its silken days and sweet breezes was still upon us as I readied myself for the days ahead with their promise of quick forays into the specialist medical community. The sun was almost ever-present and in the afternoon you could peel off the layers of clothing that were no longer necessary. The fresh, moist air of the greenhouse was filled with the fragrance of herbs and the rich, earthy aroma of wet peat moss. I learned to gauge my life by the seasons and their tempestuous churnings often mirrored my life.

There was always the work with its long, exhausting ninety-hour weeks, standing until my legs felt like stiff poles. I was in close quarters with customers pumping me for information and demanding horticultural surrender. Nature was the chief disrupter and it created the most damaging surprises and produced the most fearful stress, especially during the early spring when sudden weather changes threatened to quickly kill our carefully nurtured stock. Joyce and I talked about these things and the stress of the work and how it might cause temporary memory loss and I thought my memory problem was of a low order and was not serious.

I always believed the less I saw of doctors, the better I would be. There was a tinge of fear in me now, perhaps because I had no idea who this new doctor was and what he might find in me. I hoped it would not be a thing that had lain silent for so many years, the cancer that took my mother, or the bad heart of my father.

Having avoided doctors most of my life made them special and my lack of interaction with them meant I did not understand how they behaved. In my world doctors were receptacles of knowledge that you went to when the home medicine chest didn't work. My avoidance of the medical profession may have been part childhood fear, but the truth was that I had never needed much help from doctors. I rarely got sick, even with colds.

The doctors I have known are few, but memorable. I saw a doctor when I was a child and I can still remember the tall, youthful, balding Dr. Ashenbaugh, to whom my parents took me after we moved to Washington, DC, from Iowa. He was an old-time family practitioner, by choice, not age, and he was careful to explain things even to kids. He was always available by telephone and made occasional house calls. Once he gave me a thermometer.

It was Dr. Ashenbaugh who had come to my aid when, as a two-year-old, I got under my mother's feet in the kitchen and caused her to spill boiling spaghetti water on my back. The sweatshirt I was wearing quickly became saturated and had to be cut off my back. I carry the burn scars today. For years as a youngster, I was afraid to let any other child see me without my shirt for fear they would make fun of my scars, which were prominent, ugly disfigurements.

There was another doctor I saw just after I finished high school. A girlfriend suggested him because her mother knew him through work she did at a clinic. He was a splendid fellow and took time to tell great stories. As a young man, he had been a sailor on a cargo ship that had gone around the horn of Africa and he recounted exciting events that took place during his adventure.

While staying away from doctors had worked well over thirty years, separation from them was quickly coming to an end. I was now on the verge of seeing more doctors, nurses, and specialists than I had seen in all my previous years.

Once a disease is named, especially if it is Alzheimer's, you begin to understand it and that means recognizing it in everyday things. It is not long before you are under the spell of the disease. Its heartbeat is your heartbeat. There is danger here in trying to understand evil, especially when it is so close to you, gaining control of your brain. I worry I will become too conversant with this disease in me, and it will hijack my life with my permission.

————

Alzheimer's affects as many as four million Americans; slightly more than half of these people receive care at home, while the others are in many different health care institutions. The prevalence of Alzheimer's doubles every 5 years beyond the age of 65. Some studies indicate that nearly half of all people age 85 and older have symptoms of AD.

— "PROGRESS REPORT ON ALZHEIMER'S DISEASE," NATIONAL INSTITUTE ON AGING, 1999

I was not an immigrant like my grandfather who came with his father to America from northeastern Italy in 1892 when he was nine years old. Steamship *Werra* was slow and the food bad, he said. Going from Enrico in Italy to Harry in Iowa, he had no accent and read Shakespeare though his father took him out of sixth grade to put him to work. He and my grandmother Lottie were stuck when a Ferris wheel stalled, leaving them high above the ground. It was a perfect place for romance and soon after they married.

The cognitive changes of dementia — impairment of memory, learning, attention, and concentration — can occur in depression and make diagnosis more difficult. In general, however, a person is most likely suffering from depression if he or she has a history of psychiatric illness or has a sudden onset of cognitive symptoms, difficulties with sleep, or precipitation of symptoms by an emotional event. Also, depressed patients often complain that they're unable to concentrate or remember things, while those with dementia are generally unaware of any mental problems. For example, when depressed persons are asked a question, they are likely to say, "I don't know the answer." By contrast, someone with Alzheimer's disease might try to answer, but be unable to do so correctly.

I start thinking about something intently and then my thoughts wander through fields of memory and I bob to the surface suddenly and wonder for a moment who I am, and whether I have truly lost my mind.

———

In Alzheimer's disease, communication between some nerve cells breaks down. The destruction from Alzheimer's ultimately causes these nerve cells to stop functioning, lose connections with other nerve cells, and die. Death of many neurons in key parts of the brain

harms memory, thinking, and behavior.
— "PROGRESS REPORT
ON ALZHEIMER'S DISEASE,"
NATIONAL INSTITUTE ON AGING, 1999

Suddenly I am surrounded by clutter. I look around my room. To the right of the computer is my desk. Floating on the desk are deep piles of paper, scattered envelopes, hastily scribbled notes. File folders full of papers almost cover the telephone, the two answering machines, and the fax. A white straight-sided coffee cup with blue lettering proclaiming Lawrence Welk Resort Village is stuffed with pens and a few pencils. A wire rack designed to hold envelopes bulges with bills. A bright-red *Webster's New World Dictionary*, second college edition, leans against the fax machine. The far corner is home for racks of file folders, my last attempt to bring order on the desktop, but they are holding piles of books and random sheets of paper. On top of the pile is one of my favorite books, *My Summer in the Garden*, by Charles Dudley Warner, published in 1874. Inside the front page is an inked inscription in clear script, "Abby Bassy, July 1, 1875." It was a gift from one of my customers years ago when I was smitten with Warner's garden writing.

On my left, there is better order but there are piles of books on top of books as well. I can hardly move around the floor. I have maintained, so far, a twelve-inch-wide path in which I can see the bare, dark wooden floor.

Elsewhere there are fall garden catalogs that will eventually be mailed, four pair of leather boots, two ready to be thrown away. There is also an assortment of large, open paper bags, empty and awaiting duty. The tops of the filing cabinets are covered with stray papers and books. Notes hang from the calendar attached to the white cabinets on the wall above my desk.

There is more of this mess that need not be cataloged. This is a tragedy for a man who was once tidy but it is a snapshot of a room that mirrors my brain, a jumble of words awaiting order with nowhere to go. Meaning is lost in a hurried moment, a word lost in confusion is never recovered. So it is that Alzheimer's begins its conquest.

. . . .

The dusty, flat earth next to our apartment was perfect to catch breezes on hot evenings. Men in undershirts and slacks gathered to test horseshoe skills. My father took me to this place of competition and camaraderie. Sweat beaded on arms and chests from exertion and heat. Heavy metal horse-shoes made yellow clay smoke. A hurrah clang of metal was heard as a horseshoe slid in high for a ringer.

On March 23, 1999, I went to the National Rehabilitation Hospital for a neuro-psychological evaluation. On May 6, 1999, I underwent a full neuropsychological evalua-tion. It was numbing and took about six hours. Test results were as follows:

INTELLECTUAL: On the NART (National Adult Reading Test) which is used to estimate pre-morbid intellectual func-tioning, the patient obtained an esti-mate pre-morbid IQ score of 124 which is indicative of superior pre-morbid in-tellectual functioning.

On the WAIS-R, the patient obtained a Verbal IQ=93, a performance IQ=91 and a FSIQ=91. These scores all fall at the lower end of the range of intelli-gence classified as average. There was significant sub test variability in verbal sub test scores. On vocabulary, the pa-tient obtained an above average score. Fund of general information, digit span and verbal concept information were in the average range.

Verbal numerical reasoning was mildly impaired. On a sub test of social judgment and practical knowledge, the patient obtained a mildly to moderately impaired score. When asked what to do in the movie theater if he were the first person to notice smoke and fire, the patient responded, "yell fire." He did not know why it is better to borrow money from a bank than a friend and why a marriage license is required. On performance sub tests, the patient obtained average to low average scores on all sub tests except on picture completion on which he obtained a mildly impaired score. Picture completion requires the patient to discriminate essential from nonessential details.

— NEUROPSYCHOLOGICAL EVALUATION

Within a few months of my diagnosis, I am well aware of my cognitive loss and I can track Alzheimer's disruptive work during the day, but it is minor and subtle.

Nerve cells in the brain have the capacity to last more than 100 years.

— "PROGRESS REPORT
ON ALZHEIMER'S DISEASE,"
NATIONAL INSTITUTE ON AGING, 1999

I began writing seriously over half a lifetime ago and when I began, as a teenager on a local daily paper, I floated above the earth with excitement. With experience, I no longer floated but I was rooted to a place. I was bent on uncovering life's joys and its illusions. Now writing is like walking through a dark room. Sometimes I have to get down on my knees and crawl to find a path through the silent jungle where words are not easily picked and meaning is untrustworthy.

There are many days of elves and magic when you are small and young in the world. It is a time without routine and rules flower with baby talk, a language without lexicon, pregnant with the breath of milk and time.

———

Memory and New Learning: On the WMS-R, the patient obtained the following index scores: Verbal=54, Visual=57, Attention=88, and Delayed Recall=58. These scores are all severely impaired except for attention which is low average. The patient's recall for paragraph length story material was performed at the 2nd percentile upon immediate recall and at the first percentile upon delayed recall. Immediate recall of designs was performed at the 4th percentile and delayed recall of these designs at the first percentile.

— NEUROPSYCHOLOGICAL EVALUATION

The small white house on 14th Street was the first my parents owned after moving east. It resembled the white house left behind in Eldora but it was set at the rear of the lot and grass ran to the street where a tangle of rosebushes burst into flame in spring.

Every healthy person has 46 chromosomes in 23 pairs. Usually, people receive one chromosome in each pair from each parent. Chromosomes are rod-like structures in the cell nucleus. In each chromosome, DNA forms two long, intertwined, thread-like strands that carry inherited information in the form of genes.

— "PROGRESS REPORT
ON ALZHEIMER'S DISEASE,"
NATIONAL INSTITUTE ON AGING, 1999

Getting used to the idea of dying is difficult, emotionally and physically, but what awaits me is losing the idea of dying and that is incomprehensible and at the same time it may be liberating.

———

Neurofibrillary tangles are abnormal collections of twisted threads found inside nerve cells. The chief component of tangles is one form of the protein, tau. In the central nervous system, tau proteins are best known for their ability to bind and help stabilize micro tubules (the cell's internal support structure skeleton).

In healthy neurons, micro tubules form structures like train tracks, which guide nutrients and molecules from the bodies of the cells down to the ends of the axons. In cells affected by Alzheimer's these structures collapse. Tau normally forms the "railroad ties" or connector pieces of the micro tubule tracks. However, in Alzheimer's tau can no longer hold the railroad ties together, causing the micro tubule tracks to fall apart. The collapse of the transport system first may result in malfunctions in communication between nerve cells and later may lead to neuron death.

In Alzheimer's, chemical altered tau twists into paired helical filaments (two

threads wound around each other). These filaments are the major substance found in neurofibrillary tangles.
— "PROGRESS REPORT ON ALZHEIMER'S DISEASE," NATIONAL INSTITUTE ON AGING, 1999

. . . .

The house next door on 14th Street belonged to Mr. Rice, who had grandfatherly ways. His house was close to a street barren of sidewalks and curbs. The backyard had a large chicken house and the fence line was studded with geometrically perfect beehives. Mr. Rice often ran after his swarming bees with his net and a smoke machine. He shared honey with me.

Impressions: This fifty-seven-year-old man who subjectively reports increased word finding difficulties and forgetfulness shows neuropsychological test findings indicative of a cortical dementia and a pattern entirely consistent with early stage Alzheimer's Dementia. This patient shows impaired short term memory and poor episodic memory. He evidenced word finding difficulties both in conversation interaction and on formal testing as well as some difficulty with numerical reasoning and calculations. There is some evidence that there has been an overall intellectual functioning from pre-morbid level with the patient showing some impairment in practical and social reasoning and judgment. This pattern of deficits occurs within the context of intact ability for abstract reasoning and conceptual thought.

— NEUROPSYCHOLOGICAL EVALUATION

———

What will we do when all the lights are lit?

———

Genes are made up of four chemicals (bases) arranged in various patterns along the strands of DNA. In each gene, the bases are lined up in different order, and each sequence of bases directs the production of a different protein. Even slight changes in a gene's DNA code can make a faulty protein, and a faulty protein can lead to cell malfunction and possibly disease.

— "PROGRESS REPORT
ON ALZHEIMER'S DISEASE,"
NATIONAL INSTITUTE ON AGING, 1999

———

I am being gobbled up in time. The words are under control but the letters that form the words squirm in their own directions.

Many times I watched Mr. Rice grab a chicken by its legs and carry it to a large stump in his backyard. He threw the chicken on the stump and whacked off its head. The chicken jumped around on the grass for several minutes while blood turned its feathers red.

The large rosemary bushes were awash with blossoms, splashy blue and subtle white. These were plants beautiful to observe in the spring when winter was mild, and as I inspected their small flowers and richly aromatic foliage, I was conscious of the plant's long history of medicinal use, an irony that was not lost on me. It was said that rosemary was for remembrance.

I called the neurologist to whom my family physician referred me and made an appointment. Several weeks later, I sat in his waiting room with people I knew had to be sicker than me. They were moaning and groaning in obvious pain and discomfort. There were people on crutches and in wheelchairs. The whole place was full of the infirm, the out-of-shape, the terribly ill, and they were all much older than me or in more pain.

In comparison I looked the picture of

health and I wondered what they thought of me in their midst. If I had not been dressed so casually, they might have seen me as a salesman come to sell some ointment to the doctor. They must have wondered why I was there and that thought captured me. I was floating in a sea of doubt and I did not know what the outcome of this doctor visit would be, and that may have been the most troubling thing in my mind that afternoon.

I kept watching the clock. Waiting in a neurologist's office must be one of the modern world's more nefarious tortures. The technique of making a patient wait in a doctor's office is something that must be taught in medical school, a way to assure the patient the doctor is in charge and to telegraph how busy and important he is. It may also be a sign of how disorganized and overworked doctors are.

Finally a man in a white coat came into the waiting room and called my name. He had a hurried, brisk manner and he ushered me into a cramped, spare little office. He sat down at his desk and motioned me into a chair opposite him. The only humanizing thing in the room was a set of abstract watercolors on paper pinned to the wall next to the doctor. They turned out to be the work of his children.

The neurologist chatted for a while, outlining what he would do that day during the office visit. He began asking a few questions, gathering a wide array of personal information from me. As I talked he kept his head bowed over his notepad, writing with quick assurance, filling it with a dark, wiry scrawl.

"Mr. DeBaggio is a fifty-seven-year-old right-handed gentleman referred . . . for evaluation of memory loss," his notes say. "Patient has noted a problem with naming objects, onset about one-and-a-half years ago. Initially felt it was stress related but now is not sure. He is in the greenhouse-plant business and is having trouble remembering plants' names. Also however, may think of something that he needs in another room; may go into that room but then forgets why he went there. Believes this goes along with the naming problem."

The questioning continued for some time, covering my past medical history. The doctor learned what vitamins I took. Under family history/social history, he noted: "Married and has one son. Does not smoke. Drinks one-half glass of wine with dinner. Mother died of colon cancer and father died of heart disease."

The doctor stood up and walked over to the examining table and picked up a white hospital gown that lay there. He handed me the garment and asked me to undress and put on the gown. He left the room, saying he would return soon.

I changed into the hospital gown, a piece of clothing with which I was totally unfamiliar. It was style-less and not cut for warmth; the back was open and the room was chilled by air-conditioning. Garments like hospital gowns were undoubtedly designed to humble any person wearing them. I sat on the examining table, swinging my feet, waiting for him to return.

When the doctor returned, he asked me to stand and commenced an abbreviated physical exam. "Pleasant gentleman in no acute distress," his notes read. "Normal body habitus. Vital signs revealed a blood pressure of 140/80 with pulse of 70 and respiratory rate of 12. . . . Mental status resting revealed patient to be awake and alert."

Soon the type of questions changed direction and began to explore the workings of my mind in simple quick ways. Did I know where I was; what year was it; what month and day of the week? Then the doctor asked me to name the presidents of the United States, starting with the present officeholder and working backward; I got as far as Carter and he asked me to stop. "Simple and more complex calculations were intact," his notes say. "Could not reverse a five-letter word but could reverse a four-letter word. Short-term memory was three out of three objects immediately and one out of three objects after five minutes."

The most humiliating moment of the day occurred when I was asked to count backward from 100 by 7's. "Got serial sevens correctly back to 86," the neurologist noted, "subsequently said that he forgot what we were doing and then recalled on his own and then got serial sevens back to 58 correctly." That first tentative look at how my brain performed chilled me, no matter how much I made light of the methodology. Of course, neither of us knew for sure what caused the problems. The exercise illuminated the extent of how uncertain my memory had become and I found myself thinking I might be in deep mental trouble, but I dared not jump to conclusions quickly in a matter this serious.

There was an avoidance by the neurologist of the dreaded word "Alzheimer's" but it was clearly one of the options being considered. It was necessary, however, to search for other causes that might also produce similar conditions and he told me his secretary would get in touch with me to set up appointments with other specialists.

Later, when I read a copy of his notes, I came across what the neurologist's initial conclusion had been. It was chilling. From just a few simple tests, the neurologist wrote the impression: "Mild dementia versus age-related memory loss plus anxiety. Suspect the former, rule out the latter. Rule out treatable cause."

Dementia is a word used by specialists in this field to define loss or impairment of mental powers from organic causes, often Alzheimer's. It was clear that the doctor detected from his examination the familiar opening stages of Alzheimer's, but he wanted to rule out other causes. Somehow I remained optimistic.

Before I left the neurologist, he wrote an order for more blood to be drawn from me and I went downstairs and waited a few minutes. I was escorted into a small room and a nurse took four or five additional vials of blood.

Within a few days, the doctor's efficient secretary called to tell me she had made a series of appointments for me with specialists who met the approval of my HMO and I prepared for my round of testing.

―――

Two types of Alzheimer's exist: familial Alzheimer's, which is found in families where Alzheimer's follows a certain inheritance pattern; and sporadic (seemingly random) Alzheimer's, where no obvious inheritance pattern is seen. Because of differences in age at onset, Alzheimer's is further described as either early-onset (younger than 65 years old) or late onset (65 years or older). Early-onset Alzheimer's progresses faster than the more common, late-onset forms of Alzheimer's.

— "PROGRESS REPORT
ON ALZHEIMER'S DISEASE,"
NATIONAL INSTITUTE ON AGING, 1999

―――

I have talked to my son Francesco often about what I am going through. I realized the other day my openness may be a large problem for him. He must be troubled by what he sees happening to me, the slow march of disease that sends me stuttering for words. Yet he is quiet about it, watching me carefully, and searching inside himself for some early sign that my Alzheimer's was passed on to him.

★ ★ ★

When I shut my eyes at night, before I go to sleep, I am given what I imagine is a tour of my brain. Pictures of the day pass before my closed eyes and I am treated to an abstract phantasmagoria: bouncy colored lights, mountains in fantastic colors, pictures that resemble the landscape of the moon seen from a slow-moving vehicle. It is as if a television camera tuned in my brain to show me sights streaking across an inner sky. It is a moving canvas I see on which a painter delights in mixing colors and then throws them into my sleepy mind. Some nights the visual pyrotechnics are so strong it is difficult to get to sleep, something that has never happened to me before. Eventually the random shapes begin to take form and recognizable objects and scenes appear. I detect a story but then I may be asleep, or am I?

My family was surprised that the white house on 14th Street held wartime history. Mr. Cushman, the former owner, was an air raid warden and left his heavy white metal hat used during lights-out warnings. I never found the whistle but I was glad when the air raid warnings stopped and normalcy returned.

Almost all familial Alzheimer's known so far has an early onset, and many cases involve defects in three genes located on three different chromosomes (Chromosomes 1, 14 and 21). For example, if a person inherits one of these mutated genes from his or her father or mother, then that person is almost 100 percent certain to develop Alzheimer's at an early age.

— "PROGRESS REPORT ON ALZHEIMER'S DISEASE," NATIONAL INSTITUTE ON AGING, 1999

I am writing in a panic, racing against an insidious disease that gobbles memory and ends up destroying life.

. . . .

Joyce is much more than my wife, and always has been. Primarily she is a printmaker. As an artist, she is a trained observer; minutia sometimes appears to be her first love. She scrutinizes me now more than she did several years ago.

At times she is my translator and word finder when my mind slinks away from the job it was hired to do. At this stage in the disease, life is normal; only in subtle ways am I different than I was a few years ago.

Joyce and Francesco pick up these subtleties in a way that even friends might not. What is happening is hidden inside my brain and it will take time for it to be fully noticed.

Joyce grew up in a family of secrets and few words. She was not scared by her father's or mother's ways, but stripping to her soul in public is not her style. I am in the early stages of the disease and with few minor exceptions our lives are not much different than they were fifteen years ago. I drive the car, prepare my share of suppers, go grocery shopping, and do chores, but it would be inaccurate to say that Alzheimer's has not touched us.

The little white wooden structure next to the house became Santa's workshop during October, November, and December. My father spent most of his weekend and much time after dinner closeted in his workshop during this time. He made everything from shiny wooden blocks in a variety of shapes to a large and elaborate dollhouse. The dollhouse was for Mary Ann, for whom my father made tiny furniture and carpeted the floors. I received Tinkertoys, Erector sets, and model trains, the kind of toys introduced to a generation of boys to ignite their interest to change the world around them.

Mary Ann received baby dolls, miniature cooking utensils, and clothes made by my mother. It was during this time my father began to place large, colorful Christmas scenes on the front lawn.

A new world greets me every morning now. I will never see myself or the world the same way. I must cling to optimism and avoid depression, but today I am so shattered I can hardly hold a word, phrase, or sentence long enough to acknowledge it and put it on paper. It is as if I received a death sentence and I have to begin a circumscribed life in a prison of fear. I see myself differently, almost as if a death ray penetrated me. I look in a mirror and discover I am crying.

My father and I discovered tin juice cans neatly stacked in the white shed next to our house. We flattened them and my father took them to the grocery store to exchange for additional ration stamps.

I am still stunned by Joyce's reaction to my diagnosis. Though it is no wonder, she sprang at the doctor verbally. She heard a stranger abruptly inform her to prepare for an end to her life with me, a physically agonizing termination and brutally drawn out.

Lacking was an explanation of his conclusions, what was known and what could be done. Instead, fires of miscommunication burned out of control. Sorrow without tears is an empty emotion. A scream is worth a thousand words sometimes.

Joyce was brave with echoes of her days on picket lines, and anger filled her body with consternation. She erupted with swinging questions. She wanted explanations, not statements that the doctor didn't know the person who had conducted the tests. It wasn't that she didn't believe the tests, she wanted knowledge to give her understanding. She was not going to let this M.D. off the hook with a smile and a prescription. I watched as she swirled in early bereavement and lashed out for answers and cures that were the province of darkness.

My life was imaginative, rich, and filled with make-believe cowboys. From nearly the day I moved into the house on 14th Street in Arlington, I rode sawhorses into the dusty West. I was loaded with Western regalia, especially red bandannas. A cap gun was holstered on my thigh, and a big wide-brimmed hat kept the sun from my eyes.

This eager, athletic imaginative life was

fueled by radio programs filled with Western derring-do. Tom Mix, Tex Ritter, Hopalong Cassidy, Gene Autry, and the Lone Ranger were just a few of the fighters for law and order in that imaginative Wild West of radio drama. During the day I galloped without horse across the grass of the neighborhood, substituting my small legs for the horse's.

Soon my infatuation with cowboys languished and I jumped from the Wild West to a wider plane, intergalactic space with Captain Video.

Words slice through my mind so fast I cannot catch them and marry them to the eternity of the page. There is nothing else in my life now but this disease that leads to death. I am fixated on it, captured by it, and I can't win back my freedom.

Lives coast on memory.

It was difficult to find basics like sugar and meat in the grocery store. Bottles of real maple syrup were scarce but necessary for pancakes. One day my father took me to the grocery store and saw a friend who worked there. They talked for a moment and the friend went into the back room. He returned quickly with a bottle of maple syrup. Small things like real maple syrup built warm friendships lasting many years.

———

The use of functional magnetic resonance imaging (MRI) has enabled researchers in two new studies to gain a better understanding of how the brain creates memories . . . In one study focusing on visual memory, individuals given an MRI scan while viewing color pictures were later asked to identify which senses they recognized in a new series of pictures. The other study tested word recognition: after viewing a number of words while undergoing an MRI, subjects were asked to identify them by meaning or appearance. In both studies, the MRI scan revealed greater activity in certain regions of the brain as subjects viewed items that were later recognized.

These findings confirm that different kinds of memory are stored in different parts of the brain. Such knowledge can help explain memory formation, as well as provide insight into the processes that underlie memory disorders — which may allow scientists to identify where problems develop in the memory

process and in turn devise treatments that bypass damaged areas.
— *SCIENCE*, AUGUST 21, 1998, JOHNS HOPKINS WHITE PAPERS

———

Some days when I get out of bed, I feel I have more in common with my inscrutable cats, those noble animals who look into your eyes and appear to know everything in your soul. Sabina is in my lap now as I write. I thought I would never say such a thing, but she is as fine a companion and nurse as I know. Now she watches me carefully all night, caring for me as I had cared for her.

Several years ago she was overmedicated by a young veterinarian when he cleaned her teeth. She returned to us near death. I watched her shivering, bewildered, and frightened, hiding from us. Watching this cat struggle was as teary an event as being diagnosed with Alzheimer's.

Sabina came back from dying, a feat so powerful I still search her for signs that she might have returned from a secret world with a message of healing for me.

There are days I never expected, days of sorrows, frustration, and bewilderment.

. . . .

Friends often ask me unanswerable questions after I tell them of the Alzheimer's diagnosis. "Are you certain of the diagnosis?" "It can't be true. You look so healthy; the doctors have made a mistake."

It does look and feel like Alzheimer's in its beginning stages, but it is not something I have had before; this is no simple memory loss that rest and recreation improves. Does it matter what is causing my memory to fail me? Probably not. If all the doctors are wrong, it won't make any difference. I am going to live as long as I can; that has always been my goal. I am also a realist and I have begun to adjust my life so each day has a structure to it, and a purpose: to enjoy every minute I can and to focus on the work I love with herb plants, and with words. I want to write the truest sentences I can in the hope my words give others the sense of struggle and joy I feel.

I have wasted precious weeks trying to put the right words together to tell a story of a man entangled in his own death. I have searched for the potent words that announce my coming departure, but I cannot find them.

After I was diagnosed with Alzheimer's disease, I began to feel eleemosynary tingles.

This led me to think about becoming part of a trial group studying new Alzheimer's drugs prior to their release to the public. Maybe I have no chance of being saved by a miracle cure (the wait may be long) but loaning my diseased brain to science while it is still in my body to benefit others, including my son, might help.

I was proud of myself for having good intentions to aid humanity. I soon realized my participation in human drug trials assumed I was in the group taking the new medicine. I thought about the time I might lose to the disease if I was unlucky enough to be in the group given the placebo.

It was at this moment Rob Lively called. Rob, now a lobbyist on Capitol Hill, befriended me years ago in my garden where I sold herb and vegetable plants. Besides gardening, Rob loved bees and tried to talk me, and almost anyone who walked into the greenhouse, into raising them. His enthusiasms are legendary. He once bought a huge number of rosemary plants and had us deliver them to Capitol Hill in an attempt to win over the U.S. Congress for some arcane political point.

More recently Rob has worked with a large pharmaceutical company and I thought he might help me get in touch with companies with drug trials about to begin on Alzheimer's. Within a couple of days he and his computer uncovered a wad of trial studies, most performed locally at the National Institutes of Health. As I read through them, it became obvious it was going to take a lot of time as well as some risk. Most trials required at least a three-day hospital stay, presumably a check-in day to prepare, a second day during which the experimental drug was ingested, and a third to watch for any immediate side effects of the drug.

There were personal risks, but more important, it took a lot of time. I had a job to go to and plants to husband. I began the book to expose my inner self in words from the deepest cavities of my being to help people understand the large picture of Alzheimer's, as well as the very personal one. I decided the book was more important. It had a potentially larger impact on public awareness. I felt more comfortable with words than with doctors and scientists.

Writing sometimes becomes difficult. Words vanish before they reach the page. Most of the time the biggest drawback is my plummeting typing accuracy. So far there are few words the spell checker cannot correct.

My first barbershop haircut ended in screaming, squirming, and tears. After that experience, my father took over tonsorial matters for the next eighteen years. His greatest challenge came with the flat-top craze. He had trouble cutting hair so it stood up to plateau evenly. He eventually cut his own hair with a razor comb. After Joyce and I married, she cut my hair.

I needed no university. I learned from pebbles.

I do not want to succumb to this illness but I am powerless in its clutches. Words come when I sit down to write, but they dance away seductively, and meaning and substance disappear quickly. Of course, this is not new; such things happen many times, but before they were retrievable and now they are not.

The grapes bloomed, their soft flowers hardly visible under huge green leaves. Soon small, hard green berries formed. I watched eagerly, uncertain of their pedigree or purpose.

One Saturday my father took me to the grape arbor. He studied the vines and their deep-purple fruit. He plucked a large grape and put it in his mouth. A little of the purple juice squirted on his chin. He chewed and then he spat the purple skin on the grass. He smiled and handed me a grape.

My mother joined us in our grape picking. She put them in a large bag. That night in the kitchen I watched her clean the grapes and gently cook them to make grape juice. It immediately became my favorite drink.

I sit on our little brick patio surrounded with memories, events not yet blotted from my mind by the eager beast in my brain gobbling time in both directions. I am in a hurry to preserve as many of these memories as I can, not because they are mine, but because all of them label and characterize the time of my life. Opportunity is no longer wasted on me.

African-Americans and Hispanics are at a greater risk of Alzheimer's disease than whites, according to a new study. Researchers followed 1,079 white, African-American, and Hispanic individuals (average age 75) for five years to determine the incidence of Alzheimer's within these groups. Participants in the study were tested for the APOE gene and examined for dementia with standard diagnostic tests.

The risk of Alzheimer's in individuals possessing the APOE 4 gene was similar regardless of racial background. However, in those who did not have the APOE 4 gene, African-Americans had more than four times the risk of developing Alzheimer's as whites, and Hispanics more than two times the risk.

Established risk factors, such as education level and family history, did not account for these differing rates. The study authors suggest that, instead, previously unidentified genes or environmental factors may be responsible for the disparity. Further studies involving individuals of varied backgrounds may reveal more about the genetic and acquired risk factors for Alzheimer's.

— *JOURNAL OF THE*
AMERICAN MEDICAL ASSOCIATION,
MARCH 11, 1998,
JOHNS HOPKINS WHITE PAPERS

Memory is a mental stabilizer and without

it the mind becomes chaotic and unstruc-
tured, allowing 1999 and 1940 to merge.

Now I know how it was, Billy. I was on the other side then and I really had no idea what you were going through. I saw you striding along the street from time to time and you looked normal and cold. Several times your daughter came up to the greenhouse and after the first time I knew when I saw her what she had come to ask. The question was always the same: "Have you seen Billy? He's wandered off again." I know the police brought you home a couple of times. How frightening it must have been to be sure of your route but lose your roadmap back.

It wasn't until the first time your daughter came that I knew you had Alzheimer's. It was a strange word and I knew little about it except you. It appeared exotic but not enough to trade places. I had no idea what went on in your brain. It is different now.

There was always a sense of desperation in your daughter's voice when she came after you. And some anger. Sometimes it seemed both of you lost something dear in each other. Where were you walking, Billy? Send me a brochure. I want a good lot if there are any left.

———

More than half of individuals with Alzheimer's disease are prone to wandering. One of the most frightening — and potentially dangerous — behaviors associated with Alzheimer's, wandering can occur at any time and be triggered by any number of factors, including medications, stress, restlessness, boredom, or an impulse to repeat an old, familiar activity, such as going to work.

Patients usually do not realize they are lost, and they seldom seek help and often do not respond when addressed. Passers-by, meanwhile, may avoid them, mistakenly attributing their behavior and appearance (patients may be dressed only in a nightgown, and act confused or disoriented) to drugs or alcohol, for example. Whether patients become lost just a few blocks from home, or travel quite far, they are vulnerable to exposure to the elements, hunger, traffic, and personal injury; and all the while, their families are left frantic with worry.

To help reunite families with Alzheimer's patients who have wandered away from home, the national Alzheimer's

Association created the Safe Return program in 1993. Funded by the U.S. Department of Justice, Safe Return registers individuals with Alzheimer's into a national database and provides them with identification materials that list their medical condition and a toll-free number that anyone who finds them should call.

Since its inception, Safe Return has registered about 40,000 individuals and has safely returned about 3,000 of them. To register, contact the Alzheimer's Association, 919 N. Michigan Ave., Suite 1000, Chicago IL 60611–1676 (800) 272-3900. There are local Alzheimer's Association units throughout the nation.

— THE JOHNS HOPKINS WHITE PAPERS, "MEMORY," 1999

I always waited eagerly for the arrival of the milkman. Bottles danced in the sturdy carrier making tinkling music as he came up the long front yard. I watched him carefully, the better to imitate him delivering empty bottles in the neighborhood.

It was a time unlike today, a time of personal service. A knife sharpener drove slowly along 14th Street periodically. He struck a piece of metal with a hammer causing a sharp unique sound that said, "Knife-sharpening man." This pied piper of honed steel attracted children like lemmings.

Trash collection was twice a week. An advance man took cans to the street where a truck with several men emptied them. Behind came another man to put the cans back.

Mail was delivered once a day, but at Christmas, letters and packages were delivered twice daily. College students were enlisted to help regular carriers.

I was amazed by the world at work, and watching the goings-on ignited my imagination. Many hours were spent imitating the men I saw working.

. . . .

There are many days of tears now. Some mornings I awake and my eyes are wet. I cry, choked with emotion I cannot express. I am having trouble reading the writing I do with a pencil or pen. It used to be clear and sharp; now it wobbles and is full of uncertainty. The words come normally but the letters are sometimes not in the proper order. I spend valuable time deciphering the meaning in each letter of the alphabet until the word's meaning becomes clear. Progress is slow and I am losing time. A few months ago I had no trouble writing. I have to be careful to spell correctly but sometimes . . .

I am aware of the loss of language more than ever before. I am afraid to write because watching the words come out distorted is painful and it reveals the destructive power of the disease over which I have no control.

Now is the last best time.

In the eyes of a Midwesterner, Washington and its environs was a strange place then, with odd customs and ways of speaking that did not immediately embrace people from Iowa. It was good that the language spoken in both places was English, and my parents noticed immediately the wide differences in the way people talked and acted in this new place.

Washington was a Southern city and my father and mother were less than happy living there. After I gained some years, my father told stories about the many Italian-Americans and African-Americans hanged by the Klan in places in the South, and there was fear of lynching in parts of Iowa even. I could never understand, at any age, how a place of birth, or skin color, could mark you for death. Little attention was paid to these things when I first arrived because my world was devoted mostly to sucking and pooping and growing, and being sheltered by my parents.

Immigration is in the blood on both sides of my family. My mother's family came from Norway, a place never mentioned to me. My father let me know early that his father, Harry DeBaggio, was born in Italy and was brought to America when he was eight. He told the story often to impress upon me the remembered roots running to the past, and to reinforce the pride and difference between our family and others.

We arrived early. The waiting room was crowded, and we took seats in an area where we could see the doctors hurrying back and forth along a carpeted corridor in their white jackets. I saw my doctor a couple of times and pointed him out to Joyce. Finally he came into the waiting room and took us to his little office with his kids' paintings on the wall.

He asked us to sit down in two straight-back chairs arranged in front of his desk. He sat opposite us and held a sheaf of documents with both hands. He looked un-comfortable, almost hiding behind his papers, creating a clear separation from us. It appeared almost as if he were trying to mask his face while handing down an un-pleasant verdict, a routine that he may have developed as a way to protect his own humanity over a number of stressful years of handing out bad news.

He looked at us both uncomfortably; then he looked at me. He was quiet and controlled.

"Have you received the final report?" I asked.

"You have Alzheimer's," he said matter-of-factly.

The statement exploded in my head and I was swept with emotion and struggled to hold it beyond recognition. Before I could catch my breath, he began talking about the medicines to be prescribed for me. It was at this moment Joyce entered the con-versation. She was shocked at the manner with which the neurologist announced what amounted to a death sentence. She wanted details, understanding, some base from which to gain strength.

"How do you know?" she asked the doctor.

"We can't be sure," he said. The MRI

and the electroencephalogram (EEG) showed a normal brain, he said. Absolute certainty on the diagnosis could only come from an inspection of my brain after I died, he explained, as a stream of other experts later confirmed. It was, as another specialist put it, "a difficult diagnosis." It was difficult to tell a patient because of its shattering effect and because it was a difficult disease with which to live. It was also difficult to determine without error when Alzheimer's was really at work.

To have Alzheimer's is a humbling experience in itself, and an emotional backbreaker. At the sound of the word you become bumbling and stupid, suddenly unable to divine the simplest of life's equations, although you try to hide it with a stiff upper lip and a knowing nod. It does not help when a doctor treats it as if it were a cold. That was when Joyce exploded with a series of questions, many of them drawn from her extensive reading about the disease.

The neurologist could not hide his anger at being questioned. Joyce wanted answers and the neurologist wanted to get along with the writing of prescriptions and send me on my way. At one point he stood up, presumably so he could become a towering figure over us. But he seemed incapable of a straightforward explanation of what it all meant. Perhaps the disease and the difficulty in diagnosing it accurately caused him to hector and prevaricate and hedge. I sat watching the two of them, one asking questions, the other trying to duck straightforward answers.

Finally both the neurologist and Joyce remembered it was me who was the patient. I could no longer question the diagnosis of Alzheimer's. How could she? Yet he had already conceded he couldn't be absolutely positive of the diagnosis.

Then he looked at us both, and it felt as if he were about to discipline a couple of errant children. "Are you both together on this?" he asked.

"I'd like to get started on the treatment," I said.

He looked at Joyce. "You both have to agree with this," he said.

Joyce was angry, startled at the neurologist's unwillingness to talk to her where she hurt, and I could see she was being put in an untenable place. She wanted an explanation and he could find none other than to impute the capabilities of the person who scored the test and suggest that I go through the same tests again given by someone else, preferably someone on the university's staff.

There was a brief pause and he looked at Joyce and said, "I'm not going to write the prescriptions until you get with the program."

The neurologist wanted us together but he didn't know how to talk to Joyce and every time he spoke he pushed her away. I couldn't understand why the doctor was being so stubborn. I didn't care whether Joyce approved of my accepting the diagnosis, and I wanted to start the medications immediately, for whatever they might be worth.

"I think I'd better come back later after we have had a chance to talk this over," I told the neurologist.

He gave us an exasperated look and showed us to the door. At that moment, I think we all knew we needed a different doctor. Later I thought about the incident and I realized it must be difficult for a doctor to work with patients whose disease is essentially untreatable, a case where science has failed in understanding the secrets of the mind and body. Every new patient with the disease is a reminder of medical science's imperfection. In the face of this, it is tough to teach optimism and offer a little hope. It is inevitable that some patient's fear and anger and bewilderment will explode and have to be absorbed by the doctor, but it need not end up frustrating his ability to relieve further suffering or hamper his ability to soothe sick bodies. The best doctors I have known have a soft touch and storytelling skills that help them gain the confidence of patients. With a disease like Alzheimer's, tender, life-affirming skills are essential.

Watching Joyce's anger at the neurologist's unwillingness to speak to her with comforting words and seeing him fight back was a shattering experience for me, especially on top of the diagnosis. Alzheimer's was not one of the diseases about which I had worried. Heart attacks took my father. I tried to follow the dietary guidelines to prevent such an outcome for me. Cancer killed my mother and I ate food that would counteract its ugly trademarks. I had never had any serious illness; I was a foreigner in a doctor's office or in a hospital. It was difficult for me to accept that I now had a fatal illness for which there was no cure, only the hope that my brain's eager course of self-destruction could be slowed for a while so I could dance with life a little longer.

★ ★ ★

Every person has two APOE genes, one inherited from each parent. Alzheimer's researchers are interested in three common alleles of APOE: *2, *3, and *4. They are studying people who inherit different forms of this gene to learn more about risk factors for Alzheimer's. The relatively rare APOE *2 may protect some people against the disease; it seems to be associated with a lower risk for Alzheimer's and later age of onset. APOE *2 also appears to protect people with Down's syndrome from developing Alzheimer's-like pathology. APOE *4 is the most common version found in the general population and may play a neutral role in Alzheimer's.

— "PROGRESS REPORT
ON ALZHEIMER'S DISEASE,"
NATIONAL INSTITUTE ON AGING, 1999

This is a book about the contrast of evil and innocence in the mind of one man.

Agitation — which can include hostile, uncooperative, and excitable behavior — is a frustrating side effect of dementia that is often treated with neuroleptic and anti-psychotic drugs in nursing homes. Unfortunately, these medications often over-sedate patients and may even hasten cognitive decline. In a new study, researchers examined the effects of an anticonvulsant, carbamazepine, on the severe agitation of 51 nursing home patients (average age 86) with Alzheimer's disease, vascular dementia, or mixed dementia. About half were given a placebo and half an average of 304 mg of carbamazepine a day.

After six weeks, symptoms had improved in 77 percent of patients taking carbamazepine, compared to only 21 percent in placebo patients. . . .

Agitation should be treated initially without drugs, but if non-drug methods fail, it is important to have drug options without disabling side effects. While these results are promising, the long-term safety and effectiveness of carabamazepine have yet to be established.

— *AMERICAN JOURNAL OF PSYCHIATRY,*
JANUARY 1998,
JOHNS HOPKINS WHITE PAPERS

———

I first learned about dirt and what it did to

clothes when I played in it as a child. My mother found many opportunities to remind me of its dangers.

My father taught me the necessity of dirt, especially garden soil. We went many times to the front lawn where the spaded earth was raked smooth. In this place, he showed me how to trickle seeds in rows and cover them lightly. They sprouted to become small heads of crisp lettuce and pungent radishes to put in salads over which olive oil and vinegar were drizzled to be eaten with gusto at the evening meal.

I sit at my worktable, a still world around me, and stare at the wall, empty of decoration. I become lost in the vocabulary of silence. Thoughts squiggle and writhe into sentences that disappear before they can be acknowledged.

I want to face this disease with clarity and reality. It is hard for me to do but it is harder for Joyce and Francesco, I think. They see me differently. I see the outside world as they do, but I also see the inside, what I am thinking and feeling. I know it is difficult for them to watch me deteriorate and if I keep quiet they won't see what is really happening. I do not want to make them suffer with me but I also want them to understand the uncontrolled evil this disease represents. They must know, as others should, the destructive power of it. Although subtle in attack, Alzheimer's is the closest thing to being eaten alive slowly.

. . . .

Fall was crisply wondrous, a special time between summer heat and angry, cold winter. Apples were ripe on the two large trees in front of the house on 14th Street. Climbing to pick firm fruit was unnecessary. The apples fell of their own weight, littering the grassy lawn with the sweet smell of autumn, a scent that quickly attracted many of Mr. Rice's bees.

Most apples were wormy and bird-pecked. My mother peeled buckets of apples to make thick, aromatic sauce to put in jars for winter use. Life was exciting in the new house. I did not know my mother was pregnant and how significantly my life was about to change.

When you are very young, every day is a new adventure and memory is not a force against which the present is compared.

Should I go to some exotic place to live a short, happy life before the bumbling and forgetfulness consumes me? Perhaps Friuli, that most Eastern province of Italy where my grandfather was born. It is not likely because we now have to think of the potentially overwhelming costs of this slow-moving, disruptive, and deadly disease.

Disorder and confusion mark life's beginning and end. In between there is a blur of questions. "Who am I?" is a frequent question, expressed at first by the simple yips and shouts of a baby. Later the question becomes all-encompassing.

For me now, any question of identity becomes profound and difficult. Without memory you lose the idea of who you are. I am struggling more than ever to find answers to questions of identity. I am flooded with early memories preserved in protected places of my brain where Alzheimer's does not reign supreme. These memories become the last remnants of my search for who I am.

Am I anything without them? This question never occurred to me until a few months ago when the word Alzheimer's entered my vocabulary. It was then that questions of being took on a sinister glow. At some time in the near future, I will begin to slip out of time, casually, in small increments. I will float on a tranquil sea of memory one moment and be swept away the next by boisterous waves that leave me confused and uncertain.

There are hints every day now that it will not be long before I look but am not able to unscramble what I see, seek the simple word but be unable to write it correctly on the page. Am I anything without my memory and the simple skills of reading and writing I learned in childhood?

What better way to die than celebrating life!

I was drawn to the railroad tracks a block from the house on 14th Street. I dared to put my ear to the rails and hear trains rumble. The tracks paralleled a creek with high granite outcroppings above it, and water splashed and burbled with the tinted colors of pollution.

Trains brought coal from mountainous western Virginia where the black rock heated buildings and homes. The diesels pulled and pushed the cars with huge, trembling black machines, their slowness and weight bespeaking fearsome power. What the railroad lacked in sparkle it made up in romance for young boys.

Waiting for trains to pass, I put pennies on the rails for the heavy engines to flatten. We ran breathless to beat the train's steady, slow pace. When I tired of trains, my friends and I played on boulders above the falls, despite parental warnings to stay clear of the sharp, slippery promontory.

The railroad is memory, its right-of-way replaced by an asphalt walk. The tamed creek flows through underground pipes and occasionally appears in narrow cuts where the old railroad traveled on its way to the muscular Potomac River.

Whatever its role in Alzheimer's, the mere inheritance of an APOE *4 gene does not predict Alzheimer's with certainty; that is APOE *4 is a risk factor gene. . . . Even with current knowledge about APOE *4, scientists cannot predict whether or when any person might develop Alzheimer's, no more than a doctor can predict whether a person with high cholesterol will have a stroke. However, many researchers believe inheriting an APOE *4 gene, in association with lower memory performance in older people that gradually worsens with time, may be a predictor for who is going to develop Alzheimer's.

— "PROGRESS REPORT
ON ALZHEIMER'S DISEASE,"
NATIONAL INSTITUTE ON AGING, 1999

My disease is hard on Joyce but she tries to hide it in a routine of work and domesticity. Alzheimer's deprives us both of life. It is the most unfair thing about my predicament. We waited too long for a time of release and retirement, and to have this disease sprout in my body like a deadly, rampaging weed is shattering us both.

The weight of unhappiness falls heavier on Joyce because she counted on recapturing the pleasure and travel we postponed. Only recently, she went through the worse double sorrow and pain a daughter has when both father and mother die within a few years of each other.

We should have had fun earlier, much more of it, instead of working constantly. I should have paid more attention to Joyce's needs and desires. Instead I focused on my own dreams, leaving no time for joint leisure, travel, and reflection. Now we have my ugly, slow death to live through.

Alzheimer's has taught me it is wise to look

in the same place many times for the thing you desire.

I can't see or feel this disease entering my brain but there will come a time when not only will I be able to see it more clearly, others will see it with clarity and sadness. They will have to live through the sorrow of my decline at the same time I will no longer recognize myself. Will there be a way for me to acknowledge this without language?

———

Animals that exhibit the pathophysiology and symptoms of human disease provide a unique opportunity to investigate the causes and development of these diseases. And they can provide a safe way to test the possible treatments. In 1996 a team of researchers at the University of Minnesota in Minneapolis, supported by the National Institutes of Aging and the National Institute of Neurological Disorders and Stroke, developed a new mouse model for Alzheimer's by inserting human genes containing different mutations of amyloid precursor protein into the mouse DNA. This genetically engineered (transgenic) mouse is the first to develop learning and memory problems characteristic of Alzheimer's patients. Researchers continue to develop new transgenic mice carrying various combinations of human genes linked to Alzheimer's.

— "PROGRESS REPORT
ON ALZHEIMER'S DISEASE,"
NATIONAL INSTITUTE ON AGING, 1999

———

One part of my life is over. A new unknown life begins today, a kind of death march, although one we all take at one time or another. There are more mysteries than ever at a time when knowledge should have provided almost enough. For me, now, my focus is on the cemetery. The only question is how many months or years before I move in.

It is not often a man in my century and at my age becomes possessed in the peculiar way Alzheimer's sneaks in and begins taking over. You have to look to the Middle Ages to find cases of "possession" that parallel this disease's slow, gruesome torture. I am now a man under an indeterminate death sentence.

The brown wooden Crosley radio with its majestic cathedral shape became my imaginative link to the world. Bill Herson, the radio voice every morning, called himself "The Time Keeper." He kept the time in view, beating the rhythms of infinity to get us off to work and school.

On sick days I stayed at home where the radio was my softly worded companion as time slipped by. There was also the Breakfast Club, a variety show from Chicago, where everybody was invited to march around the breakfast table. Afternoons were devoted to steamy soap operas like Stella Dallas; this was a good time to nap.

The best part of the radio day was evening adventure serials. They lasted fifteen to thirty minutes and brought spine-tingling stories to keep listeners hanging with excitement day after day. These programs had a similar theme, the rooting out of evil, and featured stars like Johnny Dollar, Tom Mix, the Shadow, Sergeant Preston and his dog King. Classic themes of the war between good and evil filled the airwaves, preparing me for life with morality plays without nuance.

This evil disease sleeps on the edge of my consciousness, always there to remind me of its wicked strength over me.

It is in the lonely hours that words sing to me and recently they warbled of death and my obituary. What will the obituary say? Will it talk of the small, lonely boy inside the man? Will it reveal the moments of explosive emotion? Have my deepest secrets been leaked by someone I hurt? Will it spotlight my indecision? Here, have a look at my broken heart.

I have made a mess of a life designed with much promise. Instead of a glowing résumé, I have a tattered life of insignificance. A life in backroom picture frame shops and steam-hissing tailor shops. A life of dirt and exhaustion. It turns out, to my recent surprise, a life that touched a few people and made them happy, or so they say in their kind letters.

An ordinary life by definition. Just what I feared. No photos on the French Riviera surrounded by near-naked young women; just a few pieces of paper with honors from my friends. Yes, just an ordinary life; and now it is coming to an end. The finish does not feel ordinary at all. It is the most exciting time in my life. As it should be.

New findings from Finland support the theory that head injuries increase the risk for dementia. During an initial two-and-a-half year period, researchers monitored the occurrence of head injuries in 588 individuals age 70 and older, and administered a shortened version of the mini-mental state exam at the beginning and end of the study period. They then followed the subjects for another two-and-a-half years to see if cognitive decline resulted from or preceded head injuries occurring after a fall.

A major head injury — for example, one involving fractures, dislocations, or the need for stitches — more than tripled the risk of cognitive decline. Moreover, the second part of the study showed that the falls associated with head injuries resulted not from cognitive decline but mainly from increased age, use of psychotropic medications, or the presence of hypertension.

By evaluating individuals before they sustained an injury, this study differs from previous ones, which often relied on recall of past injuries to determine risk. While these results provide strong evidence that cognitive decline can result from head injuries, the possibility remains that the falls were an early manifestation of dementia. How head injury might lead to dementia is also under study.

— *NEUROLOGY*, FEBRUARY 1999,
JOHNS HOPKINS WHITE PAPERS

★ ★ ★

Having a deaf cat in the house has taught me a lot. During a violent rain, Sabina, the deaf cat, sat quietly in the kitchen while our second cat, Una, was nowhere to be seen. The rain and hail was loud and violent but Sabina remained calm and wanted to eat. Is there a lesson here for a person with Alzheimer's?

Instead of becoming emotional about me and this brain disease, if my friends thought about it, Alzheimer's could be a liberating event, freeing me to float through life and stand it on its head. Come fly with me.

The diagnosis, with little or no workable therapies to stop the disease, was a sentence of death as surely as birth is a sentence of sorrow, but more immediate.

I have only a few seconds to capture a thought before it disappears from my mind. Scraps of ideas flit like birds. This is the worst thing to happen to a writer.

One evening the hulking Crosley in the kitchen brought news that World War II was history. After dinner I marched up and down 14th Street waving a little American flag and shouting at the top of my voice,

"The war is over." We believed in our short-sightedness that war was finished for good.

I am running after thoughts all day. Ideas evaporate like snowflakes on a warm roof. A few years ago I felt normal and I was as sharp mentally as Francesco. Now I can't remember his age or do the math in my head to figure out how old he is. My mind is drifting out of control. I have to wait like a hunter to capture a thought. It is tough work all day to chase words flitting away before they anoint paper with their color.

I want to cry and I do, but it is a peculiar sound, like a man choking to death. I want to scream, but it won't come. Where did my voice go?

———

Investigators suspect that accumulation of beta-amyloid protein may be one cause of neuronal damage in Alzheimer's disease, possibly the oxidative reactions. But research into this topic is still preliminary. Now, in a new test-tube study, researchers used beta-amyloid protein for both humans and rats to study its reactions with other cell components.

Human beta-amyloid protein binds iron and copper — metals present in excess amounts in the brains of Alzheimer's patients — which leads to increased production of hydrogen peroxide. (In contrast, the rat protein does not.) Further evidence of these changes still must be seen in human studies, but if confirmed, these results represent a significant advance in the understanding of Alzheimer's. They show that beta-amyloid protein is directly responsible for oxidative damage to the neurons, and suggests a new approach to Alzheimer's treatment — finding interventions that prevent the oxidative reaction.

— *BIOCHEMISTRY*, JUNE 15, 1999, JOHNS HOPKINS WHITE PAPERS

As I sit in the waiting room of the doctor, I realize I am at the edge of failure and hope.

I have grown plants — herbs and vegetables mostly — from the time I was six, and for the last twenty-five years, commercially. As a job, this activity has allowed me a close look at the life and death of plant species. My prolonged contact with vegetative life has provided me with insight on the life and death of my own species. We scream louder.

Thyme was blooming in the garden when

testing was completed. I called the doctor's secretary to arrange an appointment I hoped would put a name on the malady that afflicted my memory. Over a period of three months, I underwent a series of tests. Some of them were in daylight, some in the dark, others in heavy, surrealistic machines.

Although I had been through the tests, I received no word on the results. In my usual offhand way, I interpreted this as a good sign. I was certain that if a brain tumor was discovered by the MRI, notification would have come immediately, and the same was true of the EEG. I had my doubts about what a series of written and oral tests could reveal. As I soon discovered, this day-long oral and written test was pivotal to the final diagnosis.

The doctor could see me May 3. Finally, I was to have the results of the examinations and tests carried out over the months of March, April, and May. I went to his office and sat again in the waiting room full of people who all appeared ill and in need of care. I waited over an hour on a beautiful sunny day. Finally I was called to the neurologist's office. We sat down opposite each other and sang each other pleasantries for a few minutes. He told me that the

MRI was normal, as was the EEG. Then there was the prolonged silence.

"Do you have the test results?" he asked.

"No," I replied. "I don't know anything about the test results. I thought you had them and were to give me the results today. No one told me I was supposed to have the test results at all." His face began to contort slightly and I could see he was becoming angry.

"I don't know who gave you the test," he said.

"I am sure your secretary knows," I said. "She made all the arrangements for the testing."

I had the list of specialists his secretary had given me and I handed it to him and showed him where the tests were given.

"Why wasn't the testing done here?" he asked.

"I assume it had something to do with my health insurance carrier," I said. "I know your secretary talked to them before she gave me the schedule."

The neurologist was exasperated now and on the edge of a big anger and he took the sheet of paper with the appointment list on it, signed by his secretary. He found the telephone number for the psychologist and dialed her number. He reached the psychologist's secretary. He was still sparking with the kind of anger that is slightly repressed. He asked when the test results would be available. He sounded rude and angry. The secretary told him the psychologist was scoring the tests as they spoke and the doctor would have the results within two days. He told her where the tests were to be sent and slammed down the phone.

He looked at me for a moment and pushed the piece of paper with the telephone numbers toward me without saying anything. His eyes continued to burn into me and he asked me to count backward from 100 by 7's. I objected mildly; I didn't understand what could be gained by the exercise but I accepted it as some kind of punishment. I struggled under the weight of tension and anger in the room but I couldn't get anywhere counting backward. The doctor told me to make another appointment; he said he would instruct his secretary to make sure I could get a quick appointment.

Two days later I called the psychologist who ordered the tests and scored them. I apologized to the secretary for the behavior of the doctor a few days earlier. She was tough and sweet and she told me the test results had been transmitted to the doctor the day after my visit. When I called the doctor's secretary later that day to make an appointment, she was expecting me. I could see the doctor the next day, May 6. I thought it was a good time to invite Joyce into the process and asked her to come with me. She was anxious to meet the doctor and learn the results of the tests.

Having a mother with a baby-swollen belly was strange and a lot to explain. For a three-year-old this was a difficult time. What I did understand was that I was suddenly expected to share.

As my mother got bigger, my father made arrangements for someone to care for me during the day while he worked and my mother was in the hospital for a week or more. My father knew a woman in the apartments from which we had recently moved who cared for children during the day and he enlisted her.

The woman taking care of me had a son about my age and we played together all day. One day we were pretending to be dogs and the play became too real. I bit his bottom and drew blood.

I was frightened and spent the rest of the

day in a corner until my father came to pick me up. He was worried about the other child and was outraged by my conduct. The boy with the bandaged butt ran around as if nothing happened.

I have no place to go now. I sit in a chair and try to capture fleeting moments of memories.

On 14th Street I began to discover the world by observing it and fingering it. There was radio, too, and it fired my imagination with stories of adventure, teaching me how to make new narratives of my own and dream myself into another world.

TO JOYCE

*I watched you sleep this morning
and I saw the past in clear colors.*

*I see you stroking the cat
on your lap and I see
the gentle, kind mother you are.*

*I see the kind woman who gives
her heart to me in this dirty
disruptive time.*

Our struggles

*are shared with many
unknown who thrash
as we do, and yelp at stars.*

*Even this sad, ugly battle
with my ailing humanity
will strengthen us
and give meaning to our life together.*

After my Alzheimer's diagnosis, my cat Sabina established a new pattern that pleases me. Each night, she sits in the upstairs hall waiting for me to go into the bedroom. After I get under the sheets, she jumps on the bed in the darkness and lies down next to me. I think she is telling me something. She remembers when she came back from death as a result of Joyce and I making her want to live. I often choke with emotion when I whisper in her deaf ears: "Cat, I watched you come back from dying." It is a good thing to remember when you are in the same circumstance.

———

Scientists engaged in the design and development of clinical trials to test potential treatments for Alzheimer's face a number of challenges. One is the need to recruit large numbers of participants — those diagnosed with Alzheimer's, those earlier in the course of the disease (before clinical diagnosis), and healthy elderly — so that the effects of the drug being tested and its safety and effectiveness can be measured with confidence. Close collaboration with existing research and treatment facilities, such as the Alzheimer's Disease Centers and Alzheimer's Disease Cooperative Study sites, help to ensure a sufficient pool of potential study participants. Recruitment strategies being developed for trials such as the Memory Impairment Study will also help to ensure strong participation.

A second challenge is the need to incorporate into study designs the special characteristics of people with Alzheimer's. In many respects — cognitively, behaviorally, psychologically, and medically — this patient population is different from patients who participate in clinical trials for other diseases. Because of their dementia, many may not even be fully aware that they are participating in clinical research. Extra care must be taken to accommodate Alzheimer's patients and protect their interests and rights. Their condition also means that family members and other care givers need to be included as full partners in the research effort if participation of the patient is to be successful.

Finally, the fact that several therapeutic drugs, such as donepezil and vitamin E, are now available to treat Alzheimer's has raised an important ethical issue about study designs in which one group of participants is given the investigational drug and the other group is given a placebo. Researchers are discussing whether this type of design should be abandoned in Alzheimer's research in favor of designs that compare new drugs against these existing therapies, or whether placebo-controlled trials should be continued because these therapies are not yet considered definitive standards of care of Alzheimer's.

— "PROGRESS REPORT
ON ALZHEIMER'S DISEASE,"
NATIONAL INSTITUTE ON AGING, 1999

———

For several days after I was diagnosed with Alzheimer's, there were flooding moments of tears. Joyce tried to comfort me with hugs and soft words.

My tears did not last but Joyce began to stay up ever later until I met her going to bed in the morning. I did not look, but I am sure her pillow was wet with her own tears.

After the initial shock there were friends to be told, especially those who worked for us. There were our relatives. And finally, all the fine people who bought plants from us over the years; I could not neglect them. I told them what was happening to me through a regular column I wrote in the fall catalog. There was a great response and I was in tears many times during those days because of their sweet thoughts and remembrances. It was a time I never expected, a period of hugs and fond wishes from people whose names I did not know.

A strange thing began to happen. Although some friends really didn't want the bad news I brought them, they sometimes felt slighted if someone told them about my predicament before I got around to informing them. It was subtle, but it was there, and I was surprised that even the timing of bad news was a way some friends judged their place on the imaginary pecking order of my friendship.

. . . .

With the war's end, automobile production resumed and life returned to normal rhythms. Our family joined the upward mobility of the middle class, spurred by postwar industrialism. Air conditioning appeared in barbershops and other stores. A glittering piece of hardware called television made its debut in middle-class households. These became the anchors of my world. The biggest changes were subtle and lasting. A simple world of struggle began to embrace complexity and comfort. One holdover of the world wars, the archaic Blue Laws, continued to close many businesses on Sunday in Virginia. The state's small-town ways still maintained racial segregation.

I have wasted precious weeks trying to put the right words together to tell a story of a man entangled helplessly in his own unwanted death. I have searched for the correct words to announce my coming demise. Why am I so preoccupied? A better approach is to get away from this storytelling and self-indulgence and go out and do something to benefit mankind. Better yet, go out and do something I have always wanted to do.

The only problem is I don't remember wanting to do anything other than water my plants and get soaked with sweat in the greenhouse and then come up to this little air-conditioned room and sit before this computer screen and tell a story that could be mine. I don't remember who I am when I write.

I often recall a thought or action a few minutes after it occurred, but a flood of memories from long ago bob from the depths and restore the present loss.

The strain of caring for a spouse with Alzheimer's disease often puts a significant burden on the caregiver that can negatively affect both his or her physical and mental health. Based on previous findings suggesting that women may feel more of a strain from caregiving than men, researchers in a new study measured the behavior and function of 37 male and 39 female Alzheimer's patients, and compared those findings to the burden reported by their respective spouses.

Female caregivers reported a 55 percent higher burden than male caregivers; correspondingly, male Alzheimer's patients had 48 percent higher scores on tests of dysfunction than female Alzheimer's patients. Behaviors that placed excess burden on the caregivers differed by gender. Women were more likely to feel burdened by aggression, while the burden in male caregivers was exacerbated by more psychotic behaviors, such as hallucinations.

Although conclusions cannot be drawn from this small study, it brings up a number of issues worthy of further examination. For example, what causes gender differences in the course of Alzheimer's, and how do these affect caregiver strain? Which behaviors are most difficult to deal with? And most importantly, it emphasizes that the needs of the caregiver must be addressed throughout the patient treatment.

— *ANNALS OF THE ROYAL COLLEGE OF PHYSICIANS AND SURGEONS OF CANADA*, FEBRUARY 1999, JOHNS HOPKINS WHITE PAPERS

My family saw our favorite films at home on a white bedsheet hung on a wall. There were films of me as a cowboy saddled on my sawhorse, and eventually films of Mary Ann, too. There were pictures shot in Iowa, especially the one with my grandfather showing off his dusty brown sedan with running boards. The scariest part was Grandpa riding a horse on a dirt road as a truck passed between him and the camera, as the film ran out.

I waited with anticipation to see the films of my parents' honeymoon. It showed the newlyweds throwing snowballs at each other. There were also scenes of my grandmother, who accompanied them. The films were relics as holy to me as any held by a church. Their rough amateurism reminded us where our hearts belonged.

As the plant-selling season ground to a halt under bright skies filled with merciless heat, the days emptied of meaning and customers. Now the days stretch through hours of boiling sun and they contain only a thin, winking purpose that some scribbles will become words to form glittering paragraphs to march into books. It is in these lonely hours that words sing to me.

My cousin called yesterday and on learning of my predicament immediately prescribed ginkgo, a tree extract. She is not a doctor but she reads widely the popular books on food and health. She is among those who view food as medicine. She said that after she took ginkgo, she always felt better. I told her my doctor also recommended it. I don't feel anything after taking individual pills or the full panoply. I don't even feel as if I am near death, although I know I have only a few years before I become a hatstand.

This conversation about pills reminded me of the relevance of small, familiar things, how they comfort and steady our lives. I read a poem by William Carlos Williams over forty years ago and it struck me the same way. It was a poem about the importance of small events. I admired it for its simple, tightly knit verse and its message. At the time, I wrote a similar poem, now lost, that won some kind of award for high-school poets.

THE LITTLE RED WAGON

So much depends upon
a red wheel barrow
glazed with rain water
beside the white chickens

— WILLIAM CARLOS WILLIAMS

I started walking again and each morning I stroll three easy, flat, familiar miles, always the same route. In the past, when I took this circuit, I came home with an invigorated mind full of the images and words eager to preserve for later use. Few memories have been freed on these walks recently.

Walking alone on quiet, dawn streets exercises my body and invigorates my mind with the world's wonders, and mankind's. I have traditionally taken paper and pen with me to report my thoughts on these sojourns, but I have added a small pocket recorder to catch flyaway words and ideas. These mornings are often full of moments of remembered elation and sorrow, the two emotions that balance memory.

I grew into a skinny kid and became the butt of jokes, tortured by children in the neighborhood who focused on my hairy arms and legs, and thin body. Older boys wrapped their hands around my wrists and bellowed about how tiny they were. They made fun of the splotchy red birthmark on my left wrist. In self-defense I wore long-sleeved flannel shirts and blue jeans year-round no matter the discomfort of summer heat.

Those early days of childish torture set me on a path of introspection. As early as age four or five I became tentative and withdrew into a world of imagination. Radio, and later television, became my rescue.

I don't know whether computers can have

Alzheimer's, but last January, while I was working on the spring plant catalog, the computer got out of hand. A little "t" showed up and began replicating itself until all the space was filled with "t's." I was afraid to use the machine for several weeks. I asked several people in computer stores what it might be and nobody could say for sure. Rather than bring the misbehaving machine in for service, I let it rest. When I finally opened up the computer to start working again, all the little "t" terrorists were gone. Too bad my brain can't be rested and return to its former self.

It was not long before my grandparents began to visit Virginia. They came to see this Eastern land and its differences, and make sure their children were not harmed by it. Soon my family was making annual sojourns to the flatlands of the Midwest.

On these summer trips to Iowa, I experienced sleeping on a moving railroad train and saw the differences in the Midwest and the East Coast. My little eyes opened in wonder at the dark, rich, flat land of Iowa and Illinois (my cousin Clark lived outside Chicago) where the corn grew so tall a three-year-old thought it reached the clouds.

I am suspended in time, hanging by a rotting thread of memory.

My grandfather thought he had retired from his restaurant but it was not to be; his daughter died suddenly, leaving two small children. I remember the night the phone call came from Grandpa. I watched my father as he listened quietly to the voice on the phone. As he cradled the phone to his ear, he was overcome with tears. I had seen anger and sorrow before but I had never seen anything like this. I had never seen an adult cry and didn't know what to make of it.

When he regained his composure, he said to my mother, "Dorothy is dead." Soon after, my grandparents moved back into town, ending their retirements, and returned to the restaurant business. They took into their home my Aunt Dorothy's husband and their two young children, Suzy and John.

Alzheimer's silently hollows the brain and fills it with death. Even memory is burned, leaving nothing to suck for internal substance.

———

Until now, scientists always thought

neurons were formed only during the fetal period and a short time after birth. Once a person had his or her full complement of neurons, that was that — the adult human body could not create new ones.

This past year, that idea changed dramatically as a result of research supported in part by the National Institute of Aging. Building on work in rodents, researchers at the Institute of Neurology, Sahlgrenska University Hospital, Goteborg, Sweden, and at the Salk Institute in La Jolla, California, discovered that the human brain does indeed retain an ability to generate neurons throughout life. In this study, cancer patients received injections of a compound called BrdU, which was used for diagnostic purposes. The BrdU-labeled neurons and glial cells grew in the hippocampal region. This meant that these adult human brains contained dividing neuronal stem cells (the specialized cells that generate neurons and glial cells).

Although more research will be necessary to understand the biological significance of these findings, they are provocative and may have an enormous impact on future aging research. By demonstrating that new neurons can be generated in the adult brain, it may now be possible to simulate intrinsic brain repair mechanisms to replace neurons and glial cells lost through age, trauma, and disease. Because Alzheimer's and Parkinson's diseases, strokes, and spinal cord injuries are all characterized by neuronal dysfunction and death, finding ways to stimulate the formation of new brain and spinal cord neurons may one day lead to novel therapeutic approaches for these and other conditions.

— "PROGRESS REPORT
ON ALZHEIMER'S DISEASE,"
NATIONAL INSTITUTE ON AGING, 1999

———

I was five when I started Catholic school. Youthful scholarship was not what won me an early start; it was the chance of birth. To start public school in those days, children had to be six years old before the end of November. My birthday is January 5th.

There was no cafeteria at St. James School and lunch was eaten at your desk. I wanted the same thing every day, two slices of white bread from the grocery store slathered with peanut butter and jelly. This sandwich was cut into four equal pieces in accordance with the directions of the nuns. The sandwich, wrapped in wax paper, went in a tin lunchbox, along with carrots carefully cut and scraped in accordance with the nuns' request. My mother poured milk into a little thermos, corked it, screwed on the metal top that doubled as a cup, and away I went.

. . . .

It is in the lonely hours that words sing to me. I have been thinking of my obituary all day, wondering what will be written, if anything. At one time in my short newspaper career, I wrote obits, as thankless a job as I ever had, but it was good training in the long run. If I write my obituary notice now I can die knowing I had the obit I thought I deserved. I may not need to jot down those few words. This book may become the longest obit ever written.

Going to school was important, I was told, but school made me anxious. St. James was many miles away and my parents did not have a car. I walked half a mile and crossed Washington Boulevard, a busy thoroughfare, to where I was picked up. After a few trial runs with my mother, I handled the walk by myself. From the boulevard, I was driven to school by strangers, a family with children from our church who lived nearby.

Once in a while I hear wind whistling through my brain.

————

Individuals who have a memory problem but who do not meet the generally accepted clinical criteria for Alzheimer's are considered to have mild cognitive impairment. They are becoming an increasingly important group for Alzheimer's researchers because it is now known that about 40 percent of them will develop Alzheimer's disease within three years.

A recent study, conducted by researchers at the Mayo Clinic Alzheimer's Disease Center in Rochester, Minnesota, broke new ground in this area by confirming that Mild Cognitive Impairment is a distinct clinical entity different from mild Alzheimer's and from normal age-related changes in memory. This study involved three groups: healthy older people, people with mild cognitive impairment, and patients with Alzheimer's.

The groups were followed over time and compared on demographic factors and on several different measures of cognitive function. Results showed that the main difference between the healthy study participants and those with mild cognitive impairment was in memory abilities. The mild cognitive impairment participants and the Alzheimer's patients had similar memory impairments, very much worse than the healthy participants, but Alzheimer's patients had other cognitive impairments as well.

Over time the cognitive performance of individuals with mild cognitive impairment declined more rapidly than that of the healthy participants and more slowly than that of Alzheimer's patients. However, some patients diagnosed with mild cognitive impairment did not progress to Alzheimer's, suggesting that the mildly impaired group is composed of two subgroups, only one of which is sure to progress to Alzheimer's.

— NATIONAL INSTITUTE ON AGING/NATIONAL INSTITUTES OF HEALTH, "1999 PROGRESS REPORT ON ALZHEIMER'S"

———

The frightening part of my walk to and from school was getting past the two dogs that waited for me at the top of Nichols Street. To a five-year-old, any barking dog, except your own, is frightening. My parents told me not to run because it excited the dogs, but when I followed their advice the dogs discovered a new way to scare me by nipping my shoes. Sometimes, when the dogs were restrained with tethers, I ran as fast as I could, making the dogs bark insanely as they tried to break their restraints.

My life has not prepared me for any medical ordeal and I am definitely not prepared for Alzheimer's. Before the bad news broke this year, the toughest medical trauma of my adult life had been a runny nose.

Although I have written the word "Alzheimer's" hundreds of times in writing this book, I cannot spell the word without looking it up; I often abbreviate it with "AD" or a long scribble. It is a fact that my handwriting, good at one time although not always careful, has begun to fall apart, and my spelling, not always accurate but decipherable, has crashed to the point neither I nor the spell-checker on the computer can divine what I wrote.

Dealing with the diagnosis is one thing;

dealing with the friends and well-wishers is another thing entirely and much more difficult.

There was a time in school when I became so frightened that I occasionally wet my pants, or worse. Rather than raise my hand and ask to go to the bathroom in front of the class, I did it where I sat. This trait did not endear me to the woman who drove me to and from school.

The stern nuns in their dark, sixteenth-century habits struck me with fear. Despite their kindness, they were demanding and they permitted no talking or squirming. I went to school there two years and happily transferred to public school in the third grade.

TO FRANCESCO

Do you remember the sweet green grass
we rolled in when you were
*   a diapered lad?*
Do you remember your first birthday
with cake on your face?
The first day in school?
The proud, nervous day you went off
*   to college?*
The way you worked with your

grandfather on the job?
And now the proud man,
the careful son,
I see struggling
with nature and the world,
worried that he may carry
* the secret clipped gene*
like the one that has claimed me more
for sorrow.

———

Although researchers theorize that antioxidants such as vitamin E may protect against memory loss, studies so far have not supported this theory. Now, new findings provide some evidence that vitamin E may be linked to memory performance. To examine the association between antioxidants and memory, investigators measured blood serum levels of various nutrients and administered health questionnaires, physical exams, and two simple tests of memory recall to 4,809 individuals (age 60 and older).

Those who scored poorly on the memory tests were at least twice as likely to have trouble eating nutritiously — either as a result of money problems or difficulty preparing meals — than those with normal memory scores. Poor memory was associated with low blood levels of vitamin E but not with other antioxidants, such as vitamin C, beta-carotene, and selenium.

The study authors theorize that their results may differ from earlier studies due to the greater ethnic diversity of their study population. Also, this study focused on memory — not on overall cognitive function, which has been the focus of earlier studies. Whether low levels of vitamin E actually precede or follow memory loss, however, requires further research.

— *AMERICAN JOURNAL
OF EPIDEMIOLOGY*, JULY 1, 1999

This is a story of a man surprised by his body and the sudden deterioration of his mind.

The woods were deep and came up to the back of our house. Thick hanging vines dangled from tree limbs, and the underbrush was dense. It was a place almost impenetrable in summer and frightening to a four-year-old. A narrow footpath, hardly discernible from the mass of dark greenery and tall trees, led into the woods.

Forays into the woods were made in the

summer at risk. My arms, legs, and face quickly blistered with poison ivy. My parents treated me with calamine lotion. So severe was my reaction to the itchy plant my parents had to use soft cloths to soak up the juices that wept from my open sores.

I learned to stay out of the woods that summer. I waited for frosts to disable the poison ivy before entering the natural dreamland in the leaf-littered forest. It was here my imagination, ignited by the cold silence, played for me as it does still.

Sometimes I go into the kitchen for a drink of water. By the time I get there I can't remember why I am there, but my body ends up at the ice machine. I stand in front of the ice machine and stare at it. From somewhere inside my head comes the message "You are in front of the ice machine because you wanted a glass of water."

At other times I can't remember why I went into the room and my body and mind are no help to me. Sometime later my mind flashes a message and I remember but it is so long ago I am no longer interested.

This has been a tough year for my cat,

Sabina. We took her to the vet to have her teeth cleaned. What we thought was a routine procedure turned into a nightmare. Along with cleaning her teeth the vet decided to remove a tooth without telling us. When we came for the cat, she had been traumatized, apparently the victim of improper use of sedatives. She nearly died, but she eventually pulled through. Now she cannot hear and only knows of your presence through vibrations in the floor, touch, or by sight. Some of her usual habits changed. She is frightened when you approach her from behind and touch her. More peculiar, however, she began to jump away from me as I approached her when she was looking at me. At first I thought my shoes upset her, but she had the same reaction when I approached with bare feet. Six months later, the Alzheimer's diagnosis was given and I wondered if Sabina sensed a change inside me and saw I carried death within me now.

———

Previous research has suggested higher levels of education may protect against cognitive decline later in life. Known as the "reverse" hypothesis of brain aging, this theory suggests that education — or what it measures — provides the brain with extra reserves that enable it to defend against the damage of dementia. Researchers in a new study theorized that if the reserve hypothesis is correct, then cognitively normal people with higher education levels may have evidence of extensive age-related brain changes without the usual accompanying dementia. For evidence of such changes, they took magnetic resonance imaging scans of 320 older, non-demented individuals (age 66 to 90).

Each year of education was associated with an increase of approximately 1.77 mL in peripheral cerebrospinal fluid volume. But despite the fact that peripheral cerebrospinal fluid volume is a marker of atrophy in the context of the brain, the subjects did not have dementia. Why education levels may help preserve cognitive function is unclear. But by studying brain structure, researchers hope to forge a greater understanding of possible causes of, and protective measures against, dementia.

— *NEUROLOGY,* JULY 13, 1999,
JOHNS HOPKINS WHITE PAPERS

———

Some days I am frightened to sit down and write, a task I have loved for forty years. I have also become more cunning and wary, characteristics I did not know three years ago. The disease is not visible to anyone but me, but I live with it and I am conscious of it in many ways. I find ways around the misspellings that litter my manuscript. At any moment I may lose my train of thought and end up losing another neurotransmitter and the story that went with it.

. . . .

It is now several months after I was diagnosed with Alzheimer's. During much of that time I have focused on my own shaky emotional state. It has been a time filled with tears and uncontrollable emotion. My throat still catches when I tell someone about my illness and what a slender chance of cure I have. I hope a bright researcher will create a cure soon enough to benefit me. I get angry, too, when I hear someone talk about this disease as if it were brought on by improper diet or behavior. I love kind souls who offer me books but this is a disease transmitted through genetic abnormalities and, as yet, it is without cure.

What I have overlooked is the effect of my illness on those around me, especially Joyce, even at this early stage when I appear quite normal. Joyce is on the edge of tears more often than I know. She is as frustrated as I am and as angry at the fates.

I have purposely stayed away from Francesco as much as possible, although it hurts me. Every time I have talked to him about how I feel and what we can do to transition the business to him, I end up choked with emotion and wet-eyed. He has to be cleansed of my emotion. He will have to take care of his mother, as well as himself and Tammy, after I die. I am afraid I may have passed the genes for this disease to him, as I think my mother or father may have unknowingly passed them on to me. The thought of having transmitted this hellish disease to someone you love is almost more than anyone can bear and it fills my eyes with tears.

Here is what life taught me. You can do all the healthy stuff touted as a way to extend your life, and you can believe in the 200-year-old human, but do not forget you had parents, men and women who were the results of centuries of genetic swapping. Some of those important codes on some of those genes can become damaged. Although it feels light, every morning you wake up with the weight of your genetic history. It is not your fault you have a battered gene that will kill you, but it is your burden now. Smugness in the pursuit of health is a risky attitude.

In summer when I was small, my family visited Eldora, Iowa, where I was born. My family stayed in an apartment above my grandfather's restaurant. My grandparents lived upstairs, too, in a separate apartment. One night I awoke to find smoke in the room and my parents hustling to get Mary Ann and me ready for a quick exit. Smoke was thick and in darkness I was disoriented and afraid. Frightened, at five years old, I wanted someone to comfort me, but there was no time; lives were in danger.

The stairway to the street was narrow, steep, and unfamiliar. I was terrified in the dark and refused to walk; I wanted to be carried. My mother had Mary Ann in her arms and my father was loaded with suitcases. It was not a time for a tantrum. My grandparents were already going down the stairs.

The smoke came from a grease fire in the kitchen of the restaurant. There was not much damage, but the smell of grease smoke lingered. For the rest of the week left of vacation, my family slept at Grandmother Davis' house a few blocks way. It was large and had a second floor with three big bedrooms.

———

It is a common misconception that tens of thousand of brain neurons die each day. Even if this notion were true, concerned individuals fail to take into account just how many cells the brain contains: approximately 100 billion. Even a loss of 100,000 neurons per day would still only represent a small percentage of mental reserves by age 70. In actuality, negligibly few neurons appear to die over a person's lifetime; however, they do shrink, which could explain some of the general slowing of mental functioning that occurs in middle or old age. Serious memory problems arising from cell death occur only when whole clusters of neurons are destroyed by major disorders such as a stroke or Alzheimer's disease.
— "JOHNS HOPKINS
WHITE PAPER, 1999,"
JOHNS HOPKINS WHITE PAPERS

———

The nearness of death sometimes brings about introspection and the desire to set things right with an apology, even small things long forgotten. My sister, Mary Ann, came halfway across the country to see me soon after she learned I had been diagnosed with Alzheimer's.

We grew up in the same houses, four years apart in age, but we have seen and heard from each other infrequently over the last thirty years. We remember who we are but we do not know each other anymore. Her three-day visit was an attempt to get in touch once more. Knowing we could never be close again, if we ever really were, I think she wanted to have one shared time that we could all remember with happiness. It turned out well but it had a surprise for me.

After her arrival with her husband, Charles, she told Joyce she wanted to see a display of photographs at the Smithsonian National Portrait Gallery in Washington, DC. The show illuminated the life of Ernest Hemingway through photographs. He was an author I was surprised to learn interested Mary Ann. Joyce thought it would be fun for all of us to go together, but Mary Ann wanted to have a day with me alone while her husband looked at investment property. This request added an unexpected sense of mystery to the visit after Mary Ann told Joyce that she wanted to be alone with me because there "were some issues that needed resolution."

Saturday morning was full of work, and as the afternoon began, Mary Ann and I were alone in the house, hunting for a morsel of food to eat before leaving for the exhibit. She stood by the stove in the kitchen, her body blocking one of the windows facing the used-car lot next door. She began to talk about long-ago events and suddenly she began apologizing to me for what happened when she was a teenager. She remembered taking my father's side against me. I no longer remembered her taking any role at all and listened politely. I remember almost none of the details except that it was during a tumultuous time after I left college a week or two after reaching the University of Arizona. I returned home, jobless, without prospects, hugging a copy of *The Catcher in the Rye*.

My father was the first person in his family to go to college and he became a lawyer. He had plans for me, always a difficult situation for a sibling, and my best hope at the time was to use my wits and ability with the English language to cause as much trouble as I could in the world. I stayed up late writing short stories and listening to clear-channel radio stations hundreds of miles away, the Hound Dog in Buffalo, New York, and especially storyteller Jean Shepherd in the Big Apple.

Every morning a copy of the *Washington Post* classified ads was on the kitchen table with large circles drawn around jobs he thought promising. It was a tough time for all of us and all our stomachs were awash with adrenaline most of the time. Eventually I found a job in a military uniform store. It provided enough money for me to leave home.

The second thing my sister wanted to apologize for was a dinner we had in her house thirty years ago. She intended to prepare the meal, but was late coming home. As it got later, Joyce and I, baby Francesco, and my mother all got hungry. In an effort to speed dinner's arrival, I began preparing it from the food I found in the kitchen. When my sister arrived she was not pleased — to put it mildly.

There were probably occasions I could have cited where I slipped and made Mary Ann's life miserable but I thought these confessions were often deathbed behaviors, necessary to make amends before shutting off the lights.

In the little Italian town of Romans de Varmo, in Friuli where my grandfather was born, the family name was Di Biasio. The birth certificates and military documents, written with flair in dark, wiry lines and with official stamps, were carefully stored in his grandfather's safe-deposit box to preserve a bit of the past. When my great-grandfather and his son, Enrico, landed on Ellis Island, an immigration officer, hearing their last name and paying no attention to their documents, wrote their names as Di Biaggio. In keeping with tradition they accepted this new appellation as their "American" name.

When Enrico, called Harry in America, became a naturalized citizen he signed the papers De Biaggio. He later "Americanized" his name, as he used to say, by eliminating the "i" between "B" and "a" in DeBiaggio. Many "American" names migrated this way.

————

Events that create a large emotional impact are usually the ones that are best remembered later. In a new study, researchers explored the connection between emotional memories and the brain's limbic system, which governs the most basic urges and emotions. They showed 10 volunteers a series of pictures: some to elicit strong emotions (both good and bad), some that were emotionally neutral, and some that were intellectually, but not emotionally, interesting. The subjects were monitored by PET scans during the viewing. Four weeks later, they were shown more pictures and asked to identify the ones they had seen.

The PET scans revealed more activity in the amygdala when the emotionally powerful images were seen again, and these images were more likely to be recognized four weeks later. These findings suggest that the amygdala is activated by emotional stimuli and that it in turn stimulates the adjacent hippocampus — the major part of the brain involved in long-term memory formation.

— *NATURE NEUROSCIENCE,*
MARCH 1999,
JOHNS HOPKINS WHITE PAPERS

———

My parents tried to instill in me a loathing for name-calling and described it to me as the verbal equivalent of spitting on someone, and I have tried to adhere to their dictum. I have recently discovered I have become a different kind of name-caller and it has come as a result of memory loss. My ability to remember words is diminishing rapidly and I can often see the subject but its name eludes me, and this makes me angry and frustrated.

Sometimes, after I finish spluttering at being unable to find the right word, I ask my companion to help me find the word and I proceed to describe in detail the object or situation the lost word means. It is always some common word and it is easily picked out by a brain not being destroyed by Alzheimer's. It has been difficult for me to resort to this method of communication, but there is little else I can do. In this way I have learned to carry on a peculiar dialog with the world and my fellow human beings. My conversation with the world, in person or through this computer, has become something like a game show or a Scrabble contest.

Grandma Davis lived alone in a two-story house in Eldora, Iowa, where my mother and my uncle, Amyer, grew up. Her husband, a lawyer, was killed by a man angry over a divorce settlement, and she raised the children alone, living on the rent of two farms she owned in the upper Midwest. During the Great Depression, she served as a house mother at Grinnell College while my mother studied to be a teacher.

The house was large, with four bedrooms, but that was only the beginning. There was a large library with a sliding door for privacy. It was filled with books and magazines behind glass. There was a big living room, and a well-appointed dining room. A huge kitchen was outfitted with an eating nook with painted wood tables and seats. Off the kitchen at one end was a narrow sewing room. All through the house were colorful hand-woven rugs made by the Indians in Arizona where my grandmother lived as a schoolteacher at the beginning of the twentieth century.

There was a curious place off the kitchen leading to the back door where there had been an old refrigerator. There was a special outside door to allow the iceman to put large pieces of ice into the refrigerator in earlier days. Pigeons roosted on the roof and contaminated the cistern, the source of water. The water turned yellow, so we always went to Grandpa DeBaggio's to bathe.

An upstairs room provided a clear view of the town clock atop the courthouse in the center of town. It counted the hours loudly and kept everyone aware of the passage of time. The clock tower was visible for miles across the flat land, a fixture I sought later when the family had a car and we drove to Iowa in the summer. Mary Ann and I strained to be first to view the happy sight of the town clock as my father's car neared the town. Eldora was a clean, dusted place in a calm world far from the secrets and fears rattling the East Coast.

Temptation is everywhere fueled by advice.

I spent most of my life in Arlington, Virginia, a sliver of land once considered for use as part of Washington, DC. It is a county without a city, George Washington's dream turned into a bedroom community.

Before my time, the county's high bluffs along the Potomac River offered an escape to cool breezes and lured sweltering city dwellers who built summer cottages. I remember as a child, there were signs of a rough past, remnants of its years as a home for farmers and bootleggers.

Arlington was changing fast as the 1940s opened, driven by an influx of government employees brought by FDR and the war. Children who went to school in the early days of the county traveled to Washington, DC. Later, in my time, we walked to the schools, many of them new.

By the time our family arrived, the railroad serving the county for years, the Washington and Old Dominion, was on its last passenger legs, crippled by the automobile and the bus — gas guzzlers that accelerated after the war. The school system was about to undergo expansion with the end of the conflagrations in Europe and the Far East.

. . . .

Paying income taxes became a major production several years ago. Personal income tax returns are complex enough, but with three additional business returns, we turned to professional help to understand it all. My happy fiscal stumbling during a routine compliance audit revealed I was no longer able to do my own taxes. The unfortunate part of this is that none of our companies make much money.

I sought wisdom and referrals and engaged a highly touted accountant. He did our taxes and saved us money. When I took our tax information to him the next year, we talked, and I mentioned that Joyce and I wanted to discuss financial aspects of our affairs with him because I had recently been diagnosed with Alzheimer's. He told me his company had just begun selling insurance. He ushered me into a conference

130

room so we could discuss the matter in private.

"Do you have insurance?" he asked after we were seated.

"No," I said. "Can you get insured for Alzheimer's?"

"How do you know you have Alzheimer's?" he asked. I explained I had been tested and the doctors were as certain as they could be, but current testing had about a 10 percent chance of failure.

"From what you have told me," he said, "it is difficult, almost impossible, to positively diagnose Alzheimer's. I think you should look at this on the bright side. When the insurance company calls and asks about your health, I don't think you have to offer them your own diagnosis. If doctors can't be absolutely certain until you are dead and autopsied, I don't see how you can be so sure."

He recommended insurance as a way to pay for nursing home care, which would make my last days more comfortable and less expensive. The way the discussion popped up made his eagerness to get me insured not unexpected, but what came next made me feel uneasy.

"After you apply for the insurance," he said, "the company will have an employee call you. I think you can truthfully tell them you are in good health. You have had some tests but they have not produced positive results. They will have to wait until you die and take a look at your brain before the doctors can be positive."

We got another accountant.

I am at the edge of uncertainty. I walk through my house where I have lived for over twenty-five years and I have the feeling sometimes I am in a motel, an unfamiliar place of transition.

In its early stages, Alzheimer's drug costs can be considerable. Thirty Aricept tablets retail for about $137 at the drugstore a few blocks from my house. As I write this, Aricept is the basic treatment for the disease, although there have been reports of improved medication on the horizon. It is fortunate I have heath insurance; I pay $10 per month.

My first doctor also prescribed vitamin E (2,000 IU per day) and ginkgo biloba (240 milligrams daily) in addition to vitamin B. These over-the-counter drugs and vitamins have limited effects depending on the individual. Despite the costs, however, there is no cure; the medicines are used to slow the onslaught of the disease, not cure it.

Costs to Alzheimer's victims often start low and spiral as the disease claims more mental territory. The Alzheimer's Association estimates that the average cost for someone with the disease per year is between $42,000 and $70,000. This adds up to a lifetime cost of about $174,000 per patient. The cost to the police to find and return a lost, wandering person, a common occurrence with Alzheimer's, is estimated to be close to $30,000. The Alzheimer's Association estimates the annual cost of the disease in the United States at between $80 billion and $100 billion.

When I go grocery shopping inevitable questions arise in my mind now that were unspoken in the past. Instead of picking items off the shelves as I used to, I now pause before I drop them in a cart. I look at the item carefully and ask, "Is this the last I will need of this?" It is a question that would never have occurred to me a few months ago, before my life was shattered with the Alzheimer's diagnosis. It is almost as if I am counting the days until I die, as if I knew the precise date and time. Of course I don't have a clue when my demise will be but, until a few days ago, I was certain I was going to die of this silent disease in six to eight years, the figure estimated for the life span of a person with familial Alzheimer's, the type I most likely have due to its early onset.

Although the thought of death has a powerful influence on my thinking these days, a vaccine study in mice has given me hope. It was the first study showing potential of reversing the destructive behavior in the brain that is the hallmark of Alzheimer's. The scientists, working for a subsidiary of Elan Pharmaceuticals, did this in a novel way, concocting a vaccine. The company's researchers used genetically altered mice so that they developed the plaque-like deposits commonly found in the brains of Alzheimer's patients, according to the *New York Times*. These deposits, amyloid plaques, are believed to cause cell death in the brain. When healthy mice were vaccinated, they grew up without developing the destructive plaques. The treatment eradicated plaques in diseased mice, improving damaged neurons. This was a strong scientific suggestion that the elusive cure for Alzheimer's may be found around the corner.

One day after finishing school at St. James, I

stood outside the building awaiting my ride. Suddenly my mother drove up in a strange-looking car I later learned was a Nash. It was a big surprise to have a car, the first my parents owned, and I was thrilled. I sat in the front seat with my mother as she drove home. There was a wonderful tree-covered incline on Washington Boulevard, and when the car came to it, I rolled down the window and stuck my head into the car's wind. I opened my mouth and tasted the beginning of a new world.

Once born we cannot escape our humanity. We have one chance to leave a word or two, a single concept that is worth a dime. For all our puny hopes and dreams and sparkling ideas, we cannot escape the forever of the cold, cold ground.

Alzheimer's burns the familiar and turns the world into an uncertain, frightening place.

A constant focus on dying has preoccupied me the last several months and it cannot be good for me. I have tried to shake this unhealthy focus but I am led to it. The numbers are there in all the books and research on Alzheimer's. I am not proud of my descent into the arms of Alzheimer's and its effect on me spreads to those I am around. I am an unhealthy influence on the lives of those I love. I have to find a way to stop moping around with thoughts of death before me. I have always known dying was what life was about and old age represents a historic effort on the part of those who reach it. A conversation about the weather, these days, is often a welcome relief from the constant focus on my health and my own morbid preoccupation with death.

I awoke this morning disoriented from the surreal dream I occupied in sleep. My back was sore and my left arm ached. In the dream, I worked for a man who employed me years ago and now, instead of an art supply store, I managed a street corner bunker from which I retailed newspapers and magazines. It was the kind of place you see in big, rundown cities except it was made of concrete slabs, turned in all sorts of directions, creating a multiplaned cityscape. It was as if I had slaved there forever, and at the same time it was all new. I was helpless there and my mind moved from my body. The only activity in this street corner bunker was to rush in and out of the surreal pile of concrete and wave newspapers at passersby. Eventually pieces of the structure disappeared. The decline continued until nothing was left and the street corner was empty. What remained was my memory of it, and I awoke fearful. Would I lose even the memory of having worked there?

I got up to describe the dream. I rarely have dreams now, or remember them, and I had an overwhelming feeling I was in an unfamiliar place, although I recognized my house. Everything was disappearing around me, sliding into the earth. I was bewildered and lost. It was then the tears came and I choked on them.

———

Scientists, ethicists, and other health professionals joined together in October of 1995 to write a public policy statement about the appropriateness of apoE testing and the role of genetic counseling for Alzheimer's. Discussions leading to the statement took place at a conference in Chicago, Illinois, sponsored by the National Institute on Aging and the Alzheimer's Association.

The public policy statement supports the use of apoE testing as a patient screening method. Conference participants said that further research and agreements about confidentiality are needed before they will recommend routine apoE testing.

— "NATIONAL INSTITUTES OF HEALTH FACT SHEET," 1999

I am breathless, choking with fear.

I wish I could say my memory loss came from having too much fun, but it doesn't seem possible; even overindulging in work doesn't rank as a cause. Bad luck gets most of the blame for what is happening to me and I don't know who to blame. The type of Alzheimer's I have affects about 1 percent of all those diagnosed with the disease and that explains why it seems so unusual for a fifty-seven-year-old man to have a disease that is more common among seventy- and eighty-year-olds.

I went to the local Alzheimer's Association office today. It is located in Fairfax County in a small high-rise building. I walked into the office, expecting a small, underused facility and discovered instead a bustling office with a large library. I wanted to look over the books for ideas and to see if any books had been written similar to what I had undertaken.

There were a lot of books but most of them were not written for the public in general, and I was happy.

I had not been in the office long before I met the woman who spoke with Joyce the day before. She was glad I came because she wanted me to meet their lobbyist, who was anxious to recruit people with Alzheimer's, and their families, to help his efforts in Richmond when the General Assembly was in session. I told him I was glad to help in any way I could. I won't be much of a poster boy for the Alzheimer's Association, but I hope I can show the legislators the disease is not always one of old age only.

———

When you are very young, you fight food almost from the time you are weaned until you leave home. You know it is necessary to eat, but you like to pick your own food. In the high chair you throw it. At the dinner table you resist it. At lunch you toss it away. Kids always anticipate what parents want them to do and surprise adults with rebellious explosions. It is a wonder the young human body survives at all.

My mother's kitchen was a clean, safe place and it always smelled of apple cider vinegar. She used it on salads, of course, but it cleaned her pots and pans, as well, when a little salt was added.

She discovered the magic to keeping her family happy at the table. She cooked exactly what we wanted, even winning us over on meatless Fridays with deeply sauced, meatless spaghetti. My father did the fancy stuff of his Italian dreams. My mother stuck to the familiar, the food she discovered her children wouldn't throw on the floor. I adored orange and onion salad with French dressing out of a bottle. Hamburger nights were also favorites when the war was over and meat was more easily obtained.

My mother was without pretense in the kitchen and in life, a characteristic I still ascribe to the ways of mid-America.

. . . .

One of the small pleasures of having any illness is the opportunity it provides to tell people about it. When there is something amiss in your life, your friends like to know and commiserate with you and this is as true of a cold as it is with something so overpowering and frightening as Alzheimer's. The support I have received has been overwhelming and I hope it keeps up. It is good to know your friends support you and will do almost anything within their powers to help.

As word worked its way through the population of my friends and acquaintances, I noticed an uncommon desire to share cures. The offer of these cures is presented with kindness. I accept them with warmth and I even try some of them. The healing advice is given with best intentions and most of it makes me smile. I do not believe in miracles and it does not bother me that I have a passel of friends who do.

The first outpouring of advice came from a well-meaning cousin who filled my mailbox with pages copied from numerous books claiming cures for Alzheimer's — from eating certain foods to exercising. Of course antioxidants are important to brain function and are contained in many foods; in fact they are part of the regimen recommended by physicians treating Alzheimer's patients, but they are not a cure.

Another friend gave me a copy of Paul Pitchford's phone-book-sized opus, *Healing with Whole Foods*. Whatever the problem, Pitchford has a cure based on eating some unappetizing food, Oriental medicine, or some unusual treatment. Ozone therapy is mentioned for use in Alzheimer's patients but it is not a cure, only a method to "improve brain function," according to Pitchford. He also blames toxic metals, especially aluminum, as a possible contributor to Alzheimer's.

A friend of nearly two decades sent me an interesting letter and gift after learning of my illness. The first object to drop from the package was a small bottle. On it were two words in large letters: "Lourdes Water." There was a picture of a supplicant and floating above her a representation of Mary. Under it was the source: "The Lourdes Bureaus, Marist Fathers, 698 Beacon Street, Boston, Mass. 02212."

My friend is known for his humorous mailings. This may have been lighthearted but I don't believe it was meant as a joke; the subject was too sensitive. The letter with the water informed me my friend's wife had a great-grandfather who had been a physician at Lourdes and helped certify miracles. A great-great-aunt of hers was in the same religious order as St. Bernadette and was present at her deathbed.

What does an atheist do with a bottle of Lourdes water, especially when the wife of the sender is so well connected? Drink the water, laugh, and thank the giver.

The day the Admiral was scheduled to arrive was filled with excitement. In my young life, this may have been the most miraculous thing to happen, and it had few rivals even later. The television came in a big, heavy box almost as tall as me. As the layers of cardboard peeled away, the glow of polished walnut came into view. In the middle was a tiny glass bubble I learned to call a "screen."

It was a large piece of furniture four feet high. The viewing screen was dwarfed by the mass of polished wood surrounding it. The monument to modernity was wrestled into a place of honor at the center of the family room and all chairs faced it.

The Admiral was the future the war postponed. My family was among the first in the neighborhood to have television. It was to change my imaginative life in ways it took years to understand.

Test patterns ruled the air waves most of the day but in the evening there was something to see — for a while. In time more movies were shown, especially during the day. Cowboy pictures from the '30s and '40s were most common but science fiction programs soon rivaled the Westerns. The images, historic and otherwise, flickering from the set primed a young boy with daydreams and imaginative play.

We are foolish, those of us who think we

can escape the traps of aging. I was one of them, dreaming of a perfect and healthy old age such as the one lived by my grandparents. Now, at fifty-eight, I realize the foolishness of my dreams, as I watch my brain self-destruct from Alzheimer's.

Following the success of the herbal memory aid ginkgo biloba, several other natural remedies with similar claims to improve mental performance have recently become available. The more prominent additions to the burgeoning market of alternative memory treatments include phosphatidylserine, vinpocetine, and huperzine A (hupA). Sold as dietary supplements, these natural agents are popping up as ingredients in a number of memory boosting products — there's even a chewing gum with added phosphatidylserine that promises to "switch on the brain." Like ginkgo, however, there is only limited evidence the newest remedies can ward off age-associated memory impairment, let alone severe dementia or Alzheimer's disease.

But at least one new agent, hupA, may stand out. Derived from the moss of *Huperzia serrata* (an herb that grows well in the outreaches of China), compounds of hupA have been used for centuries in Asia as a remedy for fever and inflammation. HupA gained increasing attention in the U.S. because it appears to have a positive effect on one of the characteristic abnormalities in Alzheimer's.

HupA has shown a positive effect in animal models, but only one small human trial has been published to date, conducted in China. Researchers randomly assigned 50 patients with mild to moderate Alzheimer's to 400 micrograms per day of purified hupA extracts for eight weeks. Another 53 subjects with roughly the same disease symptoms were given a placebo during the same period.

By the end of the study subjects who took hupA had significantly better scores on tests of memory and cognitive function than the placebo group. Overall, hupA was associated with a 58 percent improvement in symptoms, compared to 22 percent with a placebo. No serious adverse events occurred from using hupA, although the herbal remedy caused nausea, vomiting, or diarrhea in nine patients. Additional trials of hupA are currently under way.

Although hupA appears to work in a similar fashion to cholinesterase inhibitors, this does not mean that the herbal remedy is effective or safe. Only further studies can prove its usefulness. Moreover, cholinesterase inhibitors have shown only a modest effect on Alzheimer's patients, and there is no indication that this line of therapy will ultimately forestall memory loss. Even so, the proven benefits in inhibiting cholinesterase imply that hupA could have at least some therapeutic value.

— THE JOHNS HOPKINS
WHITE PAPERS, 2000

I have met, through the mail, a number of caregivers, wives, and husbands, brave men and women with hearts of gold. Their stories have a gentle, uplifting quality and I cannot let pass the story Pamela Stewart sent me.

She wrote: "As my husband, also a writer and avid reader, lost his ability to read himself, a young man named Cris, a graduate of the Iowa Writers Workshop, read aloud to him. Mark occasionally corrected his pronunciation. One day, as a joke, Cris said, 'And how do you spell that, Dr. Stewart?' To his and my astonishment, the word was spelled out correctly. Such are the quirks of this illness."

Every day is new now, with little remembrance of the day before, but with enough memory retained to know there was a yesterday. This is a new way to live and it takes getting used to.

Words, even unfamiliar ones, are more helpful now than ever before because they sometimes remind me of the past. I now lack enough mental security to be sure I remember memories of actual events; they might belong to someone else and I have stolen them for the moment, unknowingly.

I am less certain of everything, but I do not feel like a child with no history. I have a clear sense of history, I just don't know whether it is mine.

. . . .

It is now about four months since the Alzheimer's diagnosis and I remain bewildered. I do not think the Aricept, about all there is for the medical profession to prescribe, is doing much to slow my memory loss.

I started writing immediately after the diagnosis and I sense a loss in my ability to call up words on demand, and I think I have suffered some loss of vocabulary and spelling functions. Is it likely the expensive Aricept failed me? I wanted to find out what to expect from the drug and I went back to the 1999 Johns Hopkins White Paper on memory and reread the condensation from the magazine *Neurology*. In a clinical study reported in the magazine, 473 patients aged fifty and older received a placebo of 5 or 10 milligrams of Aricept, currently one of the few pharmaceuticals available. Every six weeks the patients were tested to determine whether there was any loss of memory, language, or reason. The results showed 80 percent of the Aricept patients had no cognitive loss. Among those who received no medicine, 57 percent had no memory loss. This appears to indicate the medicine was effective only 23 percent of the time.

Among those patients who had slight improvement on a single cognitive test, those ingesting the 10-milligram tablet had a slight improvement for 54 percent of the patients. At half the dose 38 percent of patients had slight improvement. Of those who got stuck with the placebo, 27 percent showed slight improvement, indicating that the large dose might account for only 27 percent effectiveness and the lower dose for only 11 percent effectiveness. In the case of slight improvement, it appears that the placebo was as effective as an expensive medicine.

Six weeks after the study's completion, the subjects were tested again. Whether the individual took the placebo or the Aricept, cognitive function scores were similar.

In a disease where small gains are important, this has some meaning but to me it is hardly a start at licking the malady. This is a big win for positive mental attitude and if that is the case, I will have to wipe the frown off my face and show my teeth more often.

My family had owned the Nash for a short time before we drove it to Iowa on a two-week summer vacation. Mary Ann was small and squirmy and sat in the back seat with my mother; I sat in front with my father. There were few motels then and my father avoided stays in people's homes that were converted into hostels. He hated the lack of privacy in such situations. He decided camping was a better, cheaper way to handle the accommodation problem. On his first camping trip my father discovered camping with two small children was the worst way to travel.

To keep Mary Ann and me content on

the long three-to-four-day drive, my mother prepared special gifts, toys designed to keep us occupied and quiet. Along with the games were stories of Iowa in the days before my birth. No matter how many games and stories were told, it was still always hot and uncomfortable.

There is a wide emotional difference between knowing you will die one day in the future and living with the knowledge you have a disease that slowly squeezes the life from you in hundreds of unexpected ways, and you have to watch it happen while those who love you stand by unable to help you.

A letter came from Maureen addressed to Joyce. It was the first time she had not telephoned me directly and I wondered what was in the letter and waited for Joyce to open it. After she read it, Joyce handed it to me. Maureen heard gossip I had Alzheimer's and she could not believe it and offered to put an end to the rumor.

I sat down and wrote to her immediately so she knew firsthand what was true. A few days later I clicked on my answering machine and Maureen's distinctive voice was talking to me and before long she was crying on the telephone. I called her back immediately but there was only an answering machine to answer her telephone. Over the next week I tried to reach her until she answered the phone and we had a nice conversation about many things and I learned she had lost several close friends in the past year, all about my age. There was great sadness in her voice and finally tears came and it was all I could do to keep from crying. It was then I realized how many people I touched in my life and how important human connection is. I once thought a person could live alone and devote a life to the mind. I outlined a play with such a theme. The main character was a man on display at a zoo. It has taken thirty years for me to realize why I couldn't finish the play.

Page one headline, *The New York Times*, October 15, 1999: "Brain May Grow New Cells Daily; Princeton Study on Monkeys Challenges Long-Held View." I wept with joy this morning when I read those words. There might be a chance for me to live. The discovery was made by Dr. Elizabeth Gould and Dr. Charles G. Gross.

"If indeed the brain is constantly renewing the cells in the cortex, hippocampus and maybe other areas," the article reported, "the prospects for learning how to repair the aged or damaged brain begin to look much more helpful. Degenerative diseases of the brain are rarely defined by loss of nerve cells." Although diseases like Parkinson's affect specific areas of the brain, it might become possible to channel new neurons into the areas of disease. "This is pie in the sky," Dr. (Eric R.) Kandel (a leading neuroscientist at Columbia University) said, "but at least there is now the possibility of thinking about it."

I hope they do a lot of fast thinking.

Going to the bank on Saturday with my father to deposit his paycheck got me thinking about money and how nice it was to earn it. At my age, this was an open invitation. A Tasty Creme doughnut route was available and I took it — going into it with early dreams in my heart.

Every Thursday the company brought boxes of doughnuts to our house. They were paid for on delivery, no return. My job was to go door-to-door selling them to neighbors. "Wanna buy some doughnuts?" was my sales pitch.

What my father and I failed to foresee was the number of glazed doughnuts the family had to eat. The neighborhood interest in doughnuts was minimal. My goal was to go to the bank with my father every week and put money into an account of my own. My father had to buy a lot of doughnuts to make that dream come true.

Alzheimer's sends you back to an elemental world before time, a world devoid of possibility and secrets. It is a world of insecurity where the certainty of words and the memory of events is unstable. It is a world of abject insecurity and tears of frustration.

I sense reality slipping away, and words become slippery sand. My life is turning into a dun-colored kaleidoscope. I think it will be only a matter of months before my life becomes a nightmare and the world becomes a freshly unknowable place where even the simplest things are difficult because they are unrecognizable.

I started three-mile daily morning walks because there is little physical exercise in writing. The walks cover familiar territory and I amuse myself trying to spot small landscape changes every day. It is a way to test and keep track of possible brain deterioration.

There is usually little to be said for the

public scribbles found on the sides of buildings and on the sidewalks, but this morning on my daily walk I came across a new one neatly engraved when the concrete was still wet on a new area of sidewalk. It is the first one I thought worthy of remembering. The lettering was careful and unhurried and it was obvious whoever wrote it thought carefully before committing to the deed. In perfectly spaced letters of knife-thin characters this artistic scofflaw wrote: "ARTISTS LIVE FOREVER." It was the first real truth I can say I have physically stumbled across.

My husband seems terrified that I am going to leave him. He says he knows he's not the man he used to be. Sometimes he berates himself, saying things like "I don't know why you would want to stay with someone like me," and in the next breath begs me to never leave. We talk about the need for reassurance and the need to make the person feel safe in the support group I attend. I need reassurance and to feel safe too. It does help to hear that his behavior, which can be so draining, is because of the Alzheimer's.

We have had a good marriage over

the years. I never dreamed I would have to spend so much time reassuring him of that. The greatest pain is that he doesn't remember so many of those special times. It is like losing a part of your history.

— C.S., FROM *LESSONS LEARNED: SHARED EXPERIENCE IN COPING*, DUKE UNIVERSITY ALZHEIMER SUPPORT GROUPS

More and more I find myself going back to books I read first twenty-five or thirty years ago. It is a weak attempt to recapture a part of my life I still want to live in me, a part of me not devoted to earth and herbs. In those long-ago days there were gardens but they were there by necessity; we needed the food.

Those were days of words and stories, paint and clay; days devoted to lovely creativity and experimentation, a time to test imagination and live in it. It was the worst of times and the best of times.

Now I wish I could have those days again in their full, expansive glory, but I am afraid to seek them because they were days of intense insecurity. That may explain why I took to books of a remembered time as a place to discover new creative energy and lost memories.

In a few minutes I can pull down from my library some of my favorite books of the era. Nearly a dozen are books by Henry Miller, many of them bought in Mexico with their fine red bindings; others I had to sneak through customs during the time Miller's books were banned in the United States: *Tropic of Cancer*, *Tropic of Capricorn*, *Black Spring*, *Sexus*, *Plexus*, *The Air-Conditioned Nightmare*, and the wonderful *Big Sur and the Oranges of Hieronymus Bosch*. There are other books such as Jack Kerouac's *On the Road* and *The Subterraneans*. All these books were hidden in my adolescent bedroom for fear my parents might find them.

There were other books, difficult and dense, *Watt* and *The Unnameable*, both by Samuel Beckett, a sly wordsmith of honor. Kenneth Patchen was another light I lingered over, especially *Sleeper's Awake* and *The Journal of Albion Moonlight*; and of course there was James Joyce's *Ulysses*, a book studied carefully; and the absurdist plays of Eugene Ionesco, which turned the world upside down. There were also the tender words of William Saroyan, an immigrant boy trying to understand a new world. I felt a kinship there I never quite understood; he wrote about me and the way I felt, and that was enough. I often revisit the political world of I. F. Stone. In the '60s he was my favorite political writer. He was a muckraker and I admired him greatly and learned much from him.

I have difficulty reading some of these books today, not because my eyes are bad or the words are so familiar but because they outline a world I never fully entered; they helped me construct a fantasy world of writing adventures. These books pleased me and educated me; they provided an adult version of childhood fantasy. After a while I was scorched by the literary heat of my book world, and I turned to the earth itself for sustenance. I found pleasure in dirt, and my creativity became crippled.

Lately I have made attempts to regain the creativity of my youth but progress is slow where the mind was once quick. There is nothing so comforting for me now as sitting in the silence of an early morning and listening to my mind spin yarns and create sentences in stories. There was no livelihood in that world of words years ago and to eat I gave it up. Those days of rich memory stayed with me and, now in my waning years, I want to return to an earlier time and join the fun and delight of a daybreak, and whistle at the moon.

It is not longing for the past from which I suffer, it is the desire to waken the person I was when I found enjoyment in artistic expression, a life I suppressed because the risks were so high.

There were many things my parents wanted to do to their new house on 14th Street. A flagstone terrace soon replaced the wooden steps as an entry to the front door. My father designed the long, wide flagstone entry and built it on weekends as I watched the new skills he possessed. I was proud of my father and went with him to the quarry in nearby Falls Church to select the large earth-colored stone.

Later he built a carport for the new Nash. It was situated to the right of the house next to the wire fence holding grapevines. For this job my father built an open wooden structure with a flat roof. He made a large wooden box and mixed the concrete in it. Each night after dinner, and on weekends all day, he hand-mixed the concrete and colored it. The carport is still there, half a century later.

I lost my driver's license Sunday. The last place I used it was a Staples store. Somewhere between the store and Monday, the brown leather billfold vanished. The process of obtaining replacements for driver's license, social security card, and medical card appeared daunting, but of course it wasn't. It took less than an hour, including travel time. Did I mention the loss of seventy-five dollars?

The episode with the missing billfold sent me into the past. As I hunted for the data required to get a replacement driver's license, I came across the two passports Joyce and I used when we went on our belated honeymoon to England the year we married, 1964. I did not immediately recognize the faces on the passports because they were so young and unmarked by time. Joyce looked into the camera with sweet assurance; her beautiful face was young and eager. It made me remember why I married her even after her mother told me she was no good. Her mother also did not want a "dirty wop" in her house.

I did not recognize myself but it must be true because my signature was above the picture. The signature had not changed markedly but the face was unknown and nearly expressionless. If there was any life in the face, it was in the dark, piercing eyes staring ahead intensely, which marked me then and now. It is a look that I have been told is evil and humorless. I had all the self-confidence of an Iowa farmer in New York City.

In youth there is little sin and I cried over the loss of innocent youth and its smooth beauty. I look in the mirror and see the tragic look of the end of life.

I have enjoyed my life but I have a nagging feeling I have not had much fun. I never slept around and got drunk; instead I read and got politicized.

I look back on my life now and see struggle and hard work sapped love of life. There is no gaiety in me now, if there ever was. I am as boring as the flat cornfields of Iowa that surrounded the little town of Eldora where I was born.

I have never been a frivolous person and I grew up believing I could change the world. Struggle, hard work, and dreams destroyed my love of life, painting, beauty, and surprise. Now I take a walk in the early misty morning dampness and I find my eyes filling with tears and grief.

My cats teach me patience. They wait silently for hours, knowing what they want — a pat under the chin, a morsel of food

— and wait for hours until they get it. What would the world be like if humans had the same approach to their lives?

Fueled by cowboy movies, pony ride rings sprouted on vacant street corners in Arlington. They were far from dusty, disorderly Westerns. For a few coins, a child was put in the saddle and a man led the pony around a small circle a few times. It was the antithesis of the open range depicted on screen and television but childish imaginations created romance from the event.

Eldora boldly called itself the pony capital of the world and my parents knew families with children and ponies. I made young Midwestern friendships with animals and kids. It was riding unlike what I experienced at home. I rode the little horses in large fenced areas in a way that inflamed my imagination — those moments still hold a sweet, full place in my memory.

I feel fine, I am not run down. If you saw me six years ago, I look the same today except for a few extra flecks of gray in my hair. I can talk while standing and I can run and jump rope.

I am dying as I write this. It is reality as

well as a mental conceit. You are reading the thoughts of a dying man. There is nothing noble or monumental I have to share with you. I can spell the word "dying" but I do not know what it really means other than the opposite of living. I have experienced living and it has already cost me many words and I have yet to understand it fully. Death is something I have never experienced. I can write the word "death" but I cannot experience it in memory as I have done all my life with other events I experienced. The thought of dying, sitting here as night approaches on this fine November day before Thanksgiving, is strange, and somehow magnificent in its own inscrutable way.

Old habits become fresh new experiences as Alzheimer's works its way through my brain.

. . . .

It has been seven months of living with the knowledge of Alzheimer's. It has done little to my life but slow it down and add some complications. I perceive some additional loss of vocabulary. Is it dangerous when nothing seems to be happening? The style of the disease is slow motion. A malady of slow, writhing death, a secret torture in the head. Being struck down suddenly with a massive heart attack is something large and earthshaking. We who suffer slowly have little to brag about when it comes time to trade illness stories.

So it is subtleties I must watch. As my vocabulary slides away ever so slowly, I do not notice it. There was a time not long ago when it was possible to feel the length and breadth of an idea or a memory. I seem to have all the time in the world to contemplate but I cannot linger over the ideas that flash through my mind now because they are quicksilver images that disappear in a flash.

I am not old enough to retire. I cannot yet be put on the disabled list. Nevertheless my eyes are feeling the heat of hell. It has been seven months since I was diagnosed with Alzheimer's and I still have not learned to live with it. Will I ever?

———

Never have I loved my husband of 41 years more than I do today, when he is so demolished by Alzheimer's that he cannot walk nor talk, cannot feed himself, cannot even shift his position in bed. What can he do? He can open his mouth when I say, "Do you want a drink?" He willingly opens his mouth when I say, "Let's brush your teeth." In fact, he even opens his mouth when he hears my voice in the hall; though he may not know I'm his wife, he does know that my presence means his favorite foods and drinks are near at hand.

Even I wonder why I can sit daily by his side as I play tapes, relate bits and pieces of news, hold his hand, tell him I love him. Yet I am content when I am with him, though I grieve for the loss of his smile, the sound of my name on his lips.

How, then, in this state of emotional bankruptcy, can I still love this man so much? Yes, he's changed; but he's still my husband. He's gentle; he's calm; he's — well, not cooperative, as that implies too active a response. But at least he passively accepts our care and attention and help.

It is said that illness is preparation for death. Surely five and a half years of existence in a nursing home should be preparation for death. I shall do nothing to prolong the miserable existence life now holds for Larry, alone, silent, isolated from people; but, oh, I

shall miss him when he is gone.
— MRS. C., *LESSONS LEARNED: SHARED
EXPERIENCES IN COPING*,
DUKE UNIVERSITY
ALZHEIMER SUPPORT GROUPS

———

My brain skitters from place to place, unable to alight on a single site that will provide me with succor or balance.

As my sister, Mary Ann, outgrew her crib, it came time for her to have a room of her own. This created a new building project for my father and he picked the summer to begin remodeling the attic. A narrow stairway already provided access. I still remember him soaking with sweat, installing the new floor and sidewalls, and covering the pitch-roof ceiling with asbestos board. He built a closet in front of the stairway.

The room had windows at either end, a ceiling so low an adult had to bend slightly to walk down the center. The roof was pitched and created walls at bed level. Two beds, one for each sidewall, were purchased from an army surplus store; a piece of plywood was placed on the springs of each bed. It was my palace as a five-year-old, the most private place in the house and in my imagination I was happy.

I am easily overwhelmed now and I am almost always on tenterhooks, ready to leap from one stone to the next in the crowded stream of consciousness.

Writing has been part of my life for over forty years. I have done it for the pure joy it brings me and to earn my bread. The best part of writing has always been shaking hands with words every day and watching stories form as a result of the handshake. I will not part with my words easily, but have little chance in this equation so stacked against me. When I am writing, I am someone else looking at me and the world.

The tough part of writing is selling it and then watching what happens. Sometimes there are big fights; rarely is there sweetness. The worst part of the writing business is waiting for the royalty check and discovering the check's so small it is not worth banking the money.

Writing is a truly liberating experience for me and I do not want to give it up. Not yet. I will keep my day job as long as I can.

In my life, I looked everywhere for the bag of sunshine but it eluded me. Now a yellow light illuminates my dreams. The yellow is deep, the color of my vitamin E capsule. Even my dreams are being attacked by Alzheimer's.

There is a dullness in my brain now to allow me to stare into silence without an idea or thought breaking the stillness.

I loved going to work with my father. No matter how occasional these visits, they were always an adventure. The day started with my mother making the sandwiches while my father and I ate breakfast. We walked to Westover by 7:30 a.m. to catch the bus to Washington.

My father made sure I had plenty to do, most of it in the art department. He brought crayons, and a stockpile of paper was available in his office. Lunch was eaten at his desk. His big swivel chair was a great adventure. The women in the office pretended to enjoy my visit.

After my mother died nearly a quarter-century later, Mary Ann came across the colorful crayon drawings she and I made working in the office. The knowledge that our parents saved this memorabilia for later times cracked my tough exterior and brought tears to my eyes, a sign that memory keeps us close to who we are as well as who we used to be.

More than ever I want to look at life without preconceptions. I want every day to be freshly watered and new but every day is filled with memories that compete with this idea of a new horizon free of the past.

I am beginning again. I am becoming again. The person I was thirty years ago was enraptured of words, real and imagined. Resily prucumbend, dilly-dolly, punk huddle. I have found the interlude wasted my memory. I am full of regrets today.

When I was six, my imaginative life was rich and filled with make-believe cowboys riding the range and intergalactic adventures in powerful airships. I am left now with dreary memories, stale words, and a life full of new mysteries.

I worked at the farm Saturday and Sunday. The day went slowly. There were not many customers for our large assortment of herbs and edible plants. It was the end of November, not a time for gardeners to be excited about planting.

I checked out a customer, something I

have done for the last twenty-five years. I was operating a cash register slightly different from those with which I am familiar. I discovered I did not know which keys to hit to complete the sale. I was embarrassed, and had to call for help. We all laughed it off.

Sometimes the kidding gets close to home. It is hard for people, even those closest to me, to understand what I am going through. They all try to understand, but losing your mind happens once a lifetime and their imaginations are lacking.

I often feel I am being treated like a child. There is a good reason for it. I am becoming a child again. Nature has turned the clock around and I am now going backward in time. It is hard to live in a grown-up body and have the mind of a child. Nobody should have to know what this is like.

Eventually, my father gave up the idea of sleeping in cars and tents on our trips to Iowa, and began the search for the perfect motel as we drove halfway across the continent. Motels were a young idea then and my father became interested in owning one. It was an idea he allowed himself to encourage. The idea of quitting his steady government job to risk everything on a motel was untypical talk.

The colorful presleep images that startled me when I first began taking Aricept are gone. They have been replaced with a raw sheet-metal color that reminds me of a trashcan. I still sleep well.

Dear Joyce,
When you can't hear my voice anymore, will you be able to feel my love?

I look in the mirror every morning and I wonder how this stranger got in the house. I have watched myself over the years, studying the effect of sun on skin but I have no idea how I really look to someone who stares into my face and watches my eyes. Will I meet a stranger on the wandering street one day and shake hands with myself?

I have shared society's fear of rats most of my life, but recently I have been inoculated with new wonder at one of nature's most ubiquitous rodents. My wavering at the unthinking hate carried for rats by the human race occurred one morning as I watched the fresh sun sparkle on the fish pools outside my window. I was nearly hypnotized by the simple spectacle nature provided in my backyard when out of the corner of my eye I saw something move. I fastened on the moving object and recognized a large gray rat at the far end of what we call the lower pool. The rat danced along the edge of the pool, darting its head into the water quickly several times, and then fled to the cover of the stone wall where it disappeared. A few moments later, the same act was repeated. His fright and hunger were palpable. I soon realized he was sharing the fish food I scattered on the water five minutes earlier. To my horror, I realized I had established a rat hotel and the dining room was now open.

Why did I feel revulsion at the rat, while I love dogs and cats, all equally human companions and scavengers? We have made cults of birds, equal in scavenging and carrying diseases. Do we not have a long history ourselves of carrying deadly diseases around the world? Humans crave intimacy and it is easily had with dogs, cats, birds, and fish. But a cantankerous rat, carrying the weight of centuries of hate and misunderstanding, becomes a target of fear. This is a fear we carry with us and perhaps it is now part of our genetic code.

What we do not understand, wild animal

or human, we fear with murderous hate and it has shaken great nations and small, and laid them waste. A disease like Alzheimer's has the same power to destroy as a bullet or a scourge, through fear and misunderstanding. Death is a natural byproduct of life and we should not fear it; we must accept it whether we call it a disease or the end of life. Now every morning I throw extra fish pellets into the lower pool for the rat.

———

Recent research suggests the tendency for Alzheimer's patients to get lost may relate to changes in the areas of the brain that interpret vision. Specifically, researchers are interested in visuospatial orientation, or how well people can perceive and interpret stimuli when they are in motion. Your ability to interpret such stimuli enables you to find your way around — for example, to follow directions or remember where you have been based on the sights you've seen. In the most recent study, investigators examined a concept called optic flow, which is the patterns of motion people see when they are moving through space. The parietal and occipital lobes of the brain process optic flow in two pathways that help orient you. You see all movement in relation to yourself by how fast they appear to be moving as you move; objects that are closer to you seem to move faster.

Researchers used computer images of moving patterns to test optic flow in 11 Alzheimer's, 12 older nondemented individuals and 6 younger nondemented individuals. They were asked, for example, to identify whether patterns of dots on the computer were moving to the left or right in one test; in another they had to identify whether the dots on the screen formed a circle or square. The Alzheimer's patients performed significantly worse on those tests than both the younger and older nondemented individuals. Spatial navigation abilities were tested directly by taking each subject on a prescribed walk and then asking them questions about the layout of the path, the directions they turned, and landmarks. Alzheimer's patients averaged only 42 percent correct responses, compared to 83 percent and 75 correct, respectively, for younger and older nondemented subjects. Moreover, poor scores on the tests of optic flow correlated with poor scores on the spatial navigation test.

That Alzheimer's affects vision and visual processing is a relatively new line of research that could have implications in the broader understanding of the disease, as well as for diagnosis and treatment. For example, it appears that abnormalities in the parietal-occipital regions of the brain cause the visual impairment. Further investigation could reveal patterns of such brain activity more fully, as well as suggest ways to prevent patients from getting lost. And, if it is an early symptom of Alzheimer's, identifying visuospatial disorientation might prove useful in diagnosis of the disease.

— THE JOHNS HOPKINS
WHITE PAPERS, 2000

I have been pondering what to do with some of my favorite things when the day arrives I can no longer use them or wonder at their beauty. I have decided to give away things I have lived with that provided me pleasure. This morning I have been looking at my collection of handmade bamboo fishing rods. I still have time to fish but for me the tackle means little. I always looked upon fishing as a sport full of lies. Not the usual lies about the number of fish or their size, but the reason for going. Going fishing has always meant getting away to some solitary place where you can be with yourself and study what being alone means. The fishing paraphernalia is camouflage for the search to find deeper meaning in life and nature.

At some point, I will no longer experience the pain of watching my mind deteriorate to a point of incomprehension. Then the loved ones around me will have the unwelcome task to look after me and shelter me from harm. My burden is slight compared to that of the truly living.

The television broadcaster started by talking about America's preparation for future wars, and just as suddenly, I recognized one of the unspoken changes in my century, the twentieth. In the early years, there was no preparation for war — there was no Pentagon, no covey of generals waiting to lead their men into battle. Now the United States is the largest vendor of military equipment and death in the world.

Trash days were treasure hunts in my neighborhood. In the summer I prowled the early-morning streets for cast-off nuggets my imagination turned to gold. Scavenging became a way of life for many of the kids in the neighborhood, much to the chagrin of parents.

One summer morning, I checked the trash as I walked up Nicholas Street. On the curb near the top of the long hill was an assortment of fine stuff put out for the trash man. The prize was a heavy, wooden-sided slot machine complete with a heavy metal handle. As I struggled to get it home, dreams of becoming rich ran through my head. At home, in my roomy attic hideaway, I inspected my fantasy. It was not quite the slot machine I observed at the Country Club in Eldora. This version was much older. Rather than a machine of chance, this was an antique candy dispenser built in the guise of a slot machine. Like its risky relative, the coin was inserted in a slot and a lever pulled, and colorful cylinders spun. Candy, not money, was the treasure to be dispensed. Unfortunately, that part of the machine was unworkable.

Like all toys, the fun soon faded and it became a large knickknack in the attic room. It was the best thing I ever acquired as trash. What made scavenging fun was its dance with chance. There was another aspect not lost on me even then. Trash put out for pickup brought me in contact with the broader world outside family and showed me history humbled.

My world has become tentative and I have difficulty naming things. It is most obvious when talking about the plants I once knew so well. Now I am full of tentativeness and my mind has become a handicap.

Having Alzheimer's helped me see how little we know ourselves, even those so well educated it is hard to understand them when they speak. No matter their station in life, almost everybody ends up asking me the same question once they know I have Alzheimer's. "Have you tried alternative medicine?" they ask. A few years ago this stuff was sold on street corners; now it is the talk of the salons. A flyer offering a pill to cure Alzheimer's arrived in the mail, probably from some well-meaning individual who wanted to offer me some hope. It was full of promise and hyperbole, but the cure recounted was from a bump on the head, not Alzheimer's.

These are drugs (when they have any active ingredients at all) for the hopeless, medicine worth a try when all else fails. It is making a lot of money for a few unscrupulous crooks who can easily delude the desperate. It is just another sign the standards we once hugged and venerated have been smashed, and true intellectual inquiry is in its coffin awaiting burial. It is dangerous and foolish to have a dual medical system.

This may be the last Christmas of which I am conscious. The sad, wide yawn of Alzheimer's releases the crushed graffiti of the soul. The graffiti will take over soon, shredding moments of lucidity, tearing them into tattered twinklings without meaning.

I was a Cub Scout without much enthusiasm for the blue uniform or what went with it. Joining the group was part of growing up, but it was not enough to keep me interested. I tired of the merit badge race quickly and my parents saw this immediately and realized I needed some other socialization method.

My Cub Scout career was not a total failure. I made a crystal radio set, the precursor to radios with vacuum tubes and speakers. Radio was still young in the late 1940s and my father remembered his own happy crystal-radio days.

I sat in the attic room overwhelmed by thoughts of invention. The crystal radio was a way to build technology skills. To construct such a thing needed little skill and the equipment was cheap: copper wire, a used oatmeal tube, some shellac, a piece of wood, and a bit of crystal.

When it was finished, I stuck the antenna out the window, slipped a cheap headset over my ears, and slowly moved a piece of copper flashing across the former oatmeal box, now circled with wire and shiny with yellow shellac. It took patience but finally I heard the lonesome twang of hillbilly music from WARL, a country music station about five miles away. I felt the warm emotion of success fill my body as I listened to sound coming through the earphone. For the first time I made real magic with my hands.

I am no longer afraid of my own vulnerability but I am also not quite used to it and am wary of its rugged power.

I can no longer remember a time when my mind held an idea for a day or two while it waited for the gestation of words that squirm across paper, alive and still malleable. Yet that time, when memory was so agreeable and sharp, was only a few years ago.

I bleed emotion every hour and play with a tricky shifting alphabet of stumbling words. I have just spent five minutes struggling to spell the word "hour."

There was crying coming from my office and I opened the door. I saw myself sitting upright in the chair, staring at the blank computer. I was crying in the dark. Will somebody help me?

Alzheimer's brings a new perspective on life. You begin to think about what the disease takes from your life. It makes you think of simple everyday things becoming difficult and then impossible.

One of the things I value most for the joy it brings is playing with my cat, Sabina.

Patients with Alzheimer's vary considerably in the clinical characteristics of their disease, including the age at which symptoms appear; the rate at which the disease progresses; the emergence of disturbances of mood, thought, perception, and behavior; the development of Parkinsonian features; and the presence of a family history of Alzheimer's-like dementia. This clinical variability suggests that Alzheimer's, as currently defined, may more closely resemble disorders such as mental retardation or anemia, which have multiple contributing causes, rather than a disease with only one cause.

In research supported by NIMH and NIA, a group of investigators at Carnegie Mellon University's Western Psychiatric Institute and Clinic are teasing out the reasons behind this clinical variability by searching for genetic and other biological factors, demographic characteristics, and environmental exposures that may influence the susceptibility of individuals to developing Alzheimer's. Identifying these risk factors will provide clues about the causes of the disease and lead to the development of effective treatments. Furthermore, because the degeneration of brain cells that leads to Alzheimer's appears to begin decades before the first symptoms emerge, risk factor profiles will be important in identifying asymptomatic individuals who are in the earliest stages of developing Alzheimer's. Such individuals are the most likely to benefit from preventive treatments.

In this research, the investigators recruited over 300 healthy first-degree relatives (brothers, sisters, or children) of patients who suffer from Alzheimer's. These relatives, who are at risk of developing Alzheimer's, were carefully evaluated for numerous characteristics that might contribute to their increased susceptibility. The study team also established a library of cell lines from most of this group so that the search for genetic and biological risk factors for Alzheimer's could continue indefinitely even after the study was concluded.

This at-risk group has now been followed for approximately 10 years and, so far, 18 have developed Alzheimer's-like dementia. As this group grows, the team will continue to search for traits that contribute to the risk of developing the disease.

The research team also has conducted studies on the brains of patients who have died with Alzheimer's to learn more about the development of depression and related behavioral disturbances in patients with dementia. These studies have shown that the death of neurons in the brain that release particular neuro-transmitters is associated with the development of serious depression (more subtle dysfunctions of these neurons may contribute to the development of clinical depression in nondemented patients). This finding may partially explain why depression in Alzheimer's is more difficult to treat with antidepressant medications. Moreover, the recurrent nature of major depression in Alzheimer's may reflect the progressive loss of these brain cells over time. Current studies are focusing on the molecular and cellular processes that lead to the death of aminergic neurons in the brains of patients with Alzheimer's as well as other aspects of the clinical biology of depression and related behavioral disturbances in Alzheimer's. Advances in this area may suggest interventions that spare these and other brain cells in Alzheimer's and other neurodegenerative disorders.

— "PROGRESS REPORT ON ALZHEIMER'S DISEASE," NATIONAL INSTITUTES OF AGING AND HEALTH, 1999

The discipline of the mind crumbles into slogans and short bursts of anger. I should run for president.

Gifts are traditional at Christmas but this year will be different. The gifts all have new meaning in the shadow of Alzheimer's. The flood of tokens and cards began early. The best so far comes from Noah and Nina. They presented me with a rock wrapped with a few strands of raffia. Their gifts are always simple and symbolic.

The heavy gray stone was plucked from a Virginia mountain stream. It is graceful and solid and it reminded me of the work of the great Italian sculptor Giacometti.

There is more to this rock than its heavy weight and solid, weathered gray appearance. It has the shape of part of a large human foot or hand. The cool, hard tactile pleasure of its bone-smooth surface invites touching. It pleases me to possess a piece of the earth blown from the ground in a fiery cloud thousands of years ago.

This coldly solid piece of the explosive past reminded me of the earth's longevity and the firmness of the past in contrast with our ephemeral present. Like many old objects it is without verbal account but nevertheless it is full of meaning and a reminder of the permanence of time. Unlike our own wispy recollections, this rock is a survivor of memories beyond our knowledge, a mute reminder that the past lives silently in the present.

Here I am alone, barking at death. Some days I feel I have fallen down a deep well of anxiety.

. . . .

Alzheimer's creates private family pain, the kind hidden and denied. It is so corrosive it can leave scars on the soul and disrupt relationships. I stepped in foolishly without a thought of the future or those around me whom I love. I believed it was my pain and I had the right to expose it, but now realize my pain has engulfed my family; my pain has become theirs.

I worry I might hurt my wife and son and engender new frustration in their lives. Joyce, Fransesco, forgive me if these revelations slap you and flavor your mourning with bitterness. Yes, with Alzheimer's mourning begins with the diagnosis. The nightmares come after the burial.

There are moments now of indecision and confusion. Before me is a cup, the same cup I have used to measure milk for my breakfast oatmeal for years. For a moment this morning I was uncertain why the cup was there or what to do with it. This is the way Alzheimer's wiggles its evil fingers at you, reminding you that before long it will have complete and absolute control over you. In many other ways the disease has come to capture my attention and barely a minute goes by that there is not a mental or physical reminder of its absolute power over me.

I am writing this while I prepare my breakfast and it is cold in the time it takes to jot these words on slips of paper I keep handy for such occasions. My crippled mind constantly sends me searching for meanings to inhabit my new life. Sometimes I think Alzheimer's is like a destructive addiction but without any pleasure accompanying it. Nobody spends money for an Alzheimer's high.

My father was a great believer in self-control. He lived by the belief that he was in control of his body. One day he came home from the office and pulled an unopened cigarette pack from his white shirt and smiled. "I didn't open this today," he said. "I am going to stop smoking because it is a bad habit."

He kept the unopened package of cigarettes in his shirt pocket for several months and eventually threw it away. I never saw him smoke a cigarette again. It was a demonstration of his willpower and his desire to cut his risk of an early death. No one knew he would be dead of heart disease before he cleared sixty.

His stern belief in willpower, seemingly such an admirable trait, brought us to loggerheads later in life when he forgot you can control yourself, but you cannot control the rest of the world.

The diagnosis was based on a six-hour test I took May 6. During those six hours, I sat at a small table answering a barrage of questions, some written, others spoken, and all designed to test my brain's function and its ability to hold thoughts and images. It was an office half the size of the neurologist's and in this office I answered questions supplied by a quiet, thoughtful woman who spent her days giving this test to scared people like me. It was a draining event both intellectually and emotionally. It was this test that produced results leading the doctors to confirm the unhappy diagnosis and I knew almost from the start I was not doing well. I had trouble remembering questions and images and words and I watched my mind grapple with things that had been without struggle only a few years ago.

The answers I gave to the questions were carefully scored as if I were in school. When I received the report from the psychologist who scored the test, I realized both she and the doctor observed clues in my behavior that alerted them to the early onset of my Alzheimer's. "The patient is a very pleasant and affable person," the psychologist wrote. "He is quite articulate but as the interview progressed, he began to experience increased word-finding difficulties."

Several weeks later, when the psychologist's assistant gave me the day-long test, she noted I was "cooperative throughout the testing and appeared to put forth maximum effort. He evidenced a marked latency to response and was slow in processing questions and instructions. He became lost in returning from the rest room to the testing room."

The report prepared by the neuropsychological evaluators minced no words, despite the accepted inconclusive method necessarily used to diagnose possible cases of Alzheimer's. "This 57 year old man," it began, "subjectively reports findings indicative of a cortical dementia and a pattern entirely consistent with early stage Alzheimer's dementia. The patient shows severely impaired short-term memory and poor episodic memory. He evidenced word finding difficulties both in conversational interaction and on formal testing, as well as some difficulty with numerical reasoning and calculations. There is some evidence that there has been a mild decline in overall intellectual functioning from a pre-morbid level with the patient showing some impairment in practical and social reasoning and judgment. This pattern of deficits occurs within the context of intact ability for abstract reasoning and conceptual thought, visuoconstructive function, and speed of information processing."

After weeks of waiting, I have been shown the test documents. I have Alzheimer's, although the doctors, skilled with their tongues and disciplined with psychiatry, are wary of making such sweeping conclusions with a disease that is notoriously difficult to diagnose in traditional ways. Instead they resort to clinical sophistry. The psychologist who scored the verbal and written tests I took wrote: "I do not believe this pattern of neuropsychological test performance can be explained solely on the basis of anxiety."

★ ★ ★

I remember being eighteen, stuck between youth and adulthood, an awful time of worry and anxiety. I was fresh from a failed attempt at college, caused by arrogance, fear, and homesickness. I spent most of the weeks at the University of Arizona pointing out "phonies," a game I picked up after becoming engrossed in J. D. Salinger's *Catcher in the Rye*. One good thing came out of my stay in Arizona — meeting Bob Hurwitt, a friend since those rough and eager days between being kids and adults. The most memorable event of that sojourn was backpacking one day in the rough mountain terrain outside Tuscon. We got lost in the evening darkness and came out of the wilderness into a chicken ranch where a farmer met us with a shotgun.

Somehow my father hoped I would matriculate at some college and I kept that idea alive by entering American University in Washington, DC. I soon ran afoul of a professor who taught modern plays. I made the unfortunate mistake of raising my hand and asking too many questions. The professor asked me to come to her office. She accused me of being a communist planted to disrupt her class. She was far too wrapped up in the make-believe of theater to have a grasp on reality so I took her advice and stayed away. Instead of attending her class I went to movies with subtitles. If I couldn't pursue my interest in European literature in school, I could get it from the movies. I also tried to keep my hand in education by attending Italian language classes in the basement of a Washington, DC, Catholic church. This satisfied my father for a while.

There is no "typical" Alzheimer's patient. There is a tremendous variability among patients in their behaviors and in their symptoms. There is no way at present to predict how quickly the disease will progress in any one person, nor predict the exact changes to occur. We do know, however, that many of these changes will present problems for the caregiver. Therefore, knowledge and prevention are the key concepts to safety.

The basic changes that will occur in Alzheimer's patients are that they will have memory problems and cognitive impairment (difficulties with thinking and reasoning), and eventually they will be unable to care for themselves. They may experience confusion, loss of judgment, and difficulty finding words, finishing thoughts, or following direction. They also may experience personality and behavior changes. For example, they may become more agitated or irritable, or very passive. Alzheimer's patients may wander from home and become lost. They may no longer be able to tell the difference between day and night, thinking that the day has just started. They may suffer from loss that affects vision, smell, or taste.

— *HOME SAFETY FOR THE ALZHEIMER'S PATIENT*, ALZHEIMER'S DISEASE RESEARCH CENTER

I remember as a teenager seeing a tall, gaunt man striding along Wilson Boulevard. He carried a briefcase and had a long gait. I saw him at various times of the day walking at different places along the highway. He was mysterious and unlike anything I had seen. Although he was quite real and looked common enough, I began to think of him as some kind of apparition.

The memory and my wonder of this anonymous man has remained with me all these years. This memory returned to me today as I walked in the early morning along my familiar route. As I walked along

I saw a man coming toward me and as he got closer I could see he was crying and his face was slicked with tears. As he passed me I looked carefully at him. He was ordinary in every respect except for tears welling from his eyes. After he was behind me, I turned for one last look at the sobbing walker, but he was not there. He seemed to have vanished as quickly as my memory. I picked up my stride and I felt tears bubbling in my eyes, obscuring my sight and wetting my face. I realized the man I had just seen crying as he walked along the sidewalk was me.

Clouded memories flit through my brain, wandering moments in a jumble of events only half-remembered. Faces smiling and sullen rise through a mist of years. Is any of this true? Can memory lie? It is too late for me to judge. Days are numb with forgetfulness and verbal stumbling.

With summers came change in the population of 14th Street and the biggest transformation occurred opposite us. An elderly couple lived there in a little rambling house with porches back and front. Except for summer the house was so quiet I hardly noticed its occupation. When summer's hot, muggy weather arrived, throngs of friends and relatives filled the house.

I sat in the front yard and watched them. To spy on them, I climbed one of the apple trees. A mysterious person showed up frequently in summer and winter. I wasn't sure whether it was a woman or a man. He seemed to have breasts like a woman, but she wore clothes like a workman's. In summer he wore undershirts like my father, the sleeveless kind, but there was the bulge of small breasts. She became an enigmatic figure to a child.

When you have a small business like ours, you come into contact with a lot of people. Many of these customers became friends over a period of time. I had no idea how many lives I touched until I wrote about myself and Alzheimer's in our little plant catalog. Soon after my self-written obituary appeared in the catalog, *Washington Post* garden columnist Adrienne Cook wrote an appreciation of my work. Soon the mail began to arrive from customers wishing me well and telling me how much plants meant to them. The mailbox overflowed in Arlington and at the Loudoun farm. I was awed. I never realized I touched people with plants and words. Nobody has so many friends and well-wishers as I.

One of my correspondents, Richard Mason, wrote me a letter full of the words of the Greek poet Hesiod and I include some of them here because I was driven by what this poet had to say so long ago. "A man may have some fresh grief over which to mourn," the poet wrote in *Theogony*, "and sorrow may have left him no more tears, but as a singer, a servant of the muses, sings the glories of ancient men and hymns to the blessed gods who dwell on Olympus, the heavy-hearted man soon shakes off his dark mood, and forgetfulness soothes his grief, for this gift of the gods diverts his mind."

My correspondent closed his letter with this thought, one easily equal to Hesiod. "For many," he mused, "Hesiod has such a bleak vision that I wonder whether I should recommend reading him to anyone. It's hard to offer comfort. What can one say in the face of misfortune? There are times when we must take root among the rocks."

I believe Hesiod would understand why I have written this book. I too have dipped my finger in grief and have been lifted by poetry.

★ ★ ★

When I was eight my parents decided to "airmail" me to Iowa to stay with my Grandmother Davis ahead of their regular vacation trip by car. The plan was for me to arrive several weeks before Mary Ann and my parents. I could help my grandmother clean her windows and cut the grass. We could get to know each other better.

I was glad to have extra time in Iowa because my grandmother had a wonderful library with the privacy of sliding doors. I was particularly looking forward to viewing her fine collection of *National Geographic* magazines, which contained extraordinary photographs of nearly naked native women around the world.

My parents worried I was too inexperienced for such a journey, never having been in an airport or on an airplane. They sought the aid of my father's cousin Pete, a military man with a family that had a long history of moving around in airplanes to different places in the world. He had relatives in Iowa and my parents thought it might be good for his son, Tex, to accompany me on the plane. Tex was six. My father talked me into believing the age difference was made up by Tex's experience.

Tickets were purchased and bags were

packed. Tex and I boarded the plane and between the stewardess and the friendly passengers we had no problems at all. We changed planes at O'Hare in Chicago and flew the short leg of the flight to Des Moines, Iowa, where all the grandparents awaited.

I went on an errand this evening soon after dark. I was sure of the direction and the route and I plodded off toward the copy store. It was a familiar location, but I had never been inside the store.

I came to an intersection at a small side street. I looked to the left and saw two cars. It appeared they were waiting for me to cross. I waited for a moment and began to cross. At that moment I looked to my left and saw a car bearing down on me. I jumped out of its way and started on. Before I crossed the street, a second car roared across the intersection, barely missing me.

Halfway to the store I had a peculiar feeling of foreboding and disorientation. It was as if I suddenly found myself in a strange city full of traps.

Finally, I came to the copy shop and it was bright and large. I walked up to a counter where a young woman waited on customers. She avoided me and would not look at me. I checked myself. My pants were zipped and there was nothing hanging from my nose. Was there something wrong? I waited. The clerk finally looked at me. She said nothing but gazed in my direction as if I were from some faraway planet. The copy machines whirred behind me. "I'd like to have this copied," I said, handing her the newspaper clipping.

"A color copy?" she asked.

"No, just black and white," I said.

"The machines are over there," she said, pointing behind me. She handed me a red card.

I went over and examined the machines. I had seen nothing like them before. They were more disorienting than walking on the sidewalk in the dark. I looked at the woman next to me. She was finishing her copying. "How does this work?" I asked her. She looked at me and there was a moment of uncertainty. "I've never used a machine like this," I said. "How do they work?"

"Put the piece to be copied in here," she said, pointing to a large opening. She walked away.

I put the clipping from the newspaper in the slot. What do I do next? I didn't have a clue. I began to feel emotional and ineffectual. I put the red piece of plastic in a slot. I pushed buttons at random. Suddenly the machine sprang to life and swished my clipping away. I lifted up a piece of metal on the other end of the machine. My clipping was lying there but no copy was to be found. I took the clipping and put it in my briefcase and walked out on to the street and went home. I can't explain why I didn't ask for help. Perhaps I was embarrassed at my sudden disability to solve minor problems. It was the first time I felt old, decrepit, and utterly useless.

On the way home, I had a peculiar feeling that the sidewalk wavered every once in a while. At intersections I was careful to look in all directions. It was a walk in which I lost something I may never get back. For a few moments, I became lost in a world I no longer recognized. Was it surrealism or Alzheiemer's? Is there any difference? It is possible I am already past the point where I can recognize either one.

This is the first time I have lost my certainty and experienced a feeling of confusion and loss, and it is frightening. Am I reaching a new stage in my life with Alzheimer's?

★ ★ ★

I am here to mourn memory.

Although my body may still be sputtering along, the day will come when I can no longer write a clear sentence and tell a coherent story. That day will be the actual time of death. The person in me who lives on until natural death occurs is only a shadow left by the deadly laugh of Alzheimer's.

———

Due to the complex changes occurring in their brain, patients with Alzheimer's may see or hear things that have no basis in reality. Hallucinations come from within the brain and involve hearing, seeing, or feeling things that are not really there. For example, patients may see children playing in the living room when no children exist.

Illusions differ from hallucinations because Alzheimer's patients are misinterpreting something that actually exists. Shadows on the wall may look like people.

Delusions are persistent thoughts that Alzheimer's patients believe are true but in reality, are not. They may be certain that someone is stealing from them, but this cannot be verified.

With all of the above symptoms, environmental adaptations may be helpful. However, if an Alzheimer's patient has ongoing disturbing hallucinations, illusions, or delusions medical evaluation is important. These symptoms may be treated with the use of medication or with advice on specific behavior management techniques.

— HOME SAFETY FOR
THE ALZHEIMER'S PATIENT,
ALZHEIMER'S DISEASE
RESEARCH CENTER

One summer, when I was eight or nine years old, I built a tree fort in the woods behind the house. It was nothing elaborate, a few boards salvaged from a moving box discovered in streetside trash and dragged home. The tree fort was little more than a platform nailed to stout tree limbs with low wooden sides around it. A series of short boards nailed to the tree trunk served as a ladder.

I was proud of the tree fort and invited two of the grandchildren who visited across the street to come and see it. The two girls were about my age, one a bit older, the other younger. I was particularly attracted to the older girl. She was not like the girls at school or in the neighborhood. Her femininity had begun to bud.

The tree fort platform was up in the leaves and there were trees all around. The three of us sat in the leafy humidity of a hot afternoon and told stories about our lives and dreams. The platform was small and we were very close and the sweat was sweet and tantalizing. I turned and my arm accidentally brushed the older girl's young, hard breasts and something strong and pleasant happened to my body and for a moment I grew larger.

The three of us played together every day, sometimes holding hands, visiting all of my favorite sites: Tommy Marshall's fine stucco clubhouse, the railroad tracks, and the creek with its large beautiful rocks.

It was in this hot, dry summer I received my first young glimmer of the secrets women and men carried that made life both rich and mysterious. I concealed my new knowledge of these things from my parents.

Doctors who treat Alzheimer's patients have the world's most thankless job. Unlike other doctors, physicians caring for those suffering from Alzheimer's have virtually no way to care for their patients. As I write, there is virtually one useful pharmaceutical available and it can only slow the onslaught of the disease for a small number of fortunate patients. These brave doctors must watch their patients' minds wither and their bodies become helpless. Sympathy and hope is almost their only tool and many of them use it well on the patient and his family. The suffering the family endures is herculean and is often the least recognized. Family members must watch as their loved one slowly disintegrates before their eyes, while they can do nothing to stop the process. For younger members of such families, there is an even greater fear — that they carry the damaged gene that triggers Alzheimer's and it will suddenly spring into action, energizing another cycle of slow, agonizing death. It is impossible to account for all the sorrow and ruined lives this disease has caused.

I awake in the morning and realize I have been crying in my sleep.

I am becoming tentative and unsure of myself. My handwriting is worse than it has ever been; I now have to print to read my writing. Instead of acquiring new knowledge, I am losing what has been stored. I regress, losing adult characteristics. I am still at the subtle stages of this decline but I feel its discomfort.

As the '50s began, my father decided to trade the old Nash for a new Ford. I went with him to buy the car. There was dickering and eventually a price was set. My father pulled out his checkbook and began to write a check for the car. The salesman became perturbed. He thought my father wanted to finance the car. It was clear financing brought more money to the dealer.

Financing was not my father's way. He was old-fashioned; he saved the money and then made the purchase. As a lawyer, he knew how to handle the salesman. My father was firm; they agreed on a price. We drove home that day in a new green Ford.

I dreamed last night of a future in which I lay in an institutional bed. I was alone in the dark room and I was beyond tears. I was tied to the bed with ropes and I was unable to move. My back and legs ached from the rigidity of my body. I lay there without memory, just a live carcass, no longer human. I was in the charnel house of dreams waiting for life to leak away and leave me still, no longer a burden.

★ ★ ★

I cannot think of death without remembering the richness and intimacy of memory.

I look around inside myself and find Alzheimer's. I am not alone. My disease touches others, some whom I know well and others I hardly recognize. This comes as something of a revelation to me. I came on this discovery by writing a farewell essay in the plant catalog we send twice a year to about 12,000 customers. So many cards and letters came from people I hardly knew and they were all telling me how sorry they were to read of my Alzheimer's. And they told me how much I meant to them over the years. I was surprised and deeply moved.

At the same time garden friends were cheering me, I realized those closest to me, Joyce and Francesco, were hurt in ways I cannot know or understand. Both of them are hesitant to reveal their inner selves and unburden their memories of the sorrow, pain, and anger. They are holding their emotions in the secret places of their hearts where silence becomes comfort. Of course, they are angry at me. I am screwing up their lives and dreams. Joyce deferred so many dreams in deference to me. She has in this decade alone suffered through the slow deaths of her parents and gone through screaming nights of pain and confusion with her taciturn mother. And then had to deal with the chaotic aftermath with secret tears. And just when things were looking better Ol' Mr. Alzheimer's hit me. No wonder her creativity has gone sour and her desire to create beauty is crippled.

Francesco, a bright man with a rich mind, is approaching his forties, and he is bowled over with secret anxiety over whether he carries the genes for Alzheimer's inherited from me. This is not the way any of us dreamed our lives. I am the luckiest of this threesome because I have found a way to use my frailties and illness to create a story that others will read and, perhaps, act on. I can open my heart and touch others to expand their lives and enrich their minds with human emotion. I am afraid we are so hurt and scared we fill ourselves with secrets to protect what is left of ourselves.

I can only guess what Joyce and Francesco are going through and it is probably not good for me to write these words to others, but they will have the opportunity to revise and extend their remarks before you read this. Alzheimer's hit them as surely as it has hit me. They are reluctant to reveal their pain and fear to me but every time they see me or talk to me they must be reminded of their own sorrow and fear. Although we try to avoid talking about Alzheimer's, I know it is on the edge of their thoughts every day, as it is mine.

Now I am asking them to do the impossible, join me on National Public Radio with Noah Adams and, with me, bleed their secret emotions in public. I love them so for acceding to this ordeal for me and for others suffering from Alzheimer's so that their suffering and confusion can be seen and named. It is in this way I hope to liberate my family from the noose I put around our lives and emotions. I have not forgotten it could also destroy us.

We try to block our fears and sorrow, hiding them in places we never go, hoping they are sequestered well enough to keep them from eating us alive. No matter how carefully we handle all this, when I die, part of them will die too. If it works as I hope, they will also find themselves reborn and reinvigorated.

The only time I feel alive now is when I am writing, under the spell of work and memories.

Walter Reed elementary school in Westover expanded rapidly after the war and I found myself in the fourth grade and in a very unlikely place, a Baptist Church annex the county rented until a new school was built. It was here a small generation learned of fear and I lost myself in art.

I spent much of my time in class drawing cartoon strips of adventurers flying to Mars and the moon. Spelling was my least favorite subject and I dreaded the Friday test days, although my father worked hard Thursday after dinner, helping me prepare for the exam.

One Friday before the spelling test, a teacher hurried into the room and talked quietly to my teacher. I heard them talking about a man with a gun who was hunting his wife who had come to see the minister at the church about marital problems. The police were already on the scene and they wanted the children out of the school-rooms and out in the open far away from the delicate confrontation in the church basement next door.

My class and all the others in the makeshift school were marched on the flat, dirt recess playground. We stood in long, quiet lines with fear and giggles flashing across our faces. Soon the man with the gun was taken away and we returned shivering to our classrooms in the church annex.

Moments of death float in my memory. My mother sucking a sliver of ice, struggling to look at me and smile as her last days approached in the tiny hospital in Eldora. In the same hospital, I watched Grandma DeBaggio die in the same ignominious way. Every time I entered the small room she shared, she struggled to raise her head and called to me in a stuttering iambic pentameter, "Tom, Tom, Tom," as if it were a chant to protect her, or was it me she sheltered with a charmed dirge? But the last breath came to her, too. There was no more chant; even my name could not protect her at 104.

. . . .

Tammy and Francesco found a wonderful little restaurant in Manassas and they took us there. I had remembered Manassas from my high-school days when it was talked about as one of the last best places to buy moonshine. Now it has changed; it is just another bedroom community. The restaurant is wedged into a strip shopping center.

Panino is a perfect name for it and it was like walking into a Fellini movie, complete with a dwarf serving tables and high-school students on prom night. The food was light-hearted and was the equal of that of a fine little trattoria.

Air raid drills were regular routines while I was in public school in the Baptist Church annex. There was claustrophobic fear, stirred by the government, that Russia was going to bomb the United States, especially Washington, DC, and its environs. At school we practiced getting under our desks. Even the smallest students wondered how the desk was going to protect us from radio-active rain and all the other fears.

At home my parents took no precautions, but the memory of the last war was still raw and real. My father told the family one night at dinner he might have to go to a secret place in the Blue Ridge Mountains where there were underground offices to house the government and operate during any wartime emergency.

Temptation is everywhere, even when you are dying.

. . . .

If there is any question that *Homo sapiens* are

animals, consider what happens to them on cloudy days. I am sitting at my desk on the second day of gray overcast and rain. I am dry and warm and the lights are on in the room but there is an unnerving feeling inside me that prevents me from doing anything. I sit and dream, a stance known to many of us on days like this. I am empty and I cannot get cranked up. My mind crawls around in the dark, unable to cough up inspiration, and I sit here waiting for something to energize me. I will have to make the best of it and wait for the sun to shine to lift my spirit. I think I can make it down to the kitchen for a sandwich; I am already over an hour late and my stomach is talking to me.

The reader is cautioned that memory often does not distinguish between fiction and the facts that have been lovingly remembered.

Imagination is surely an important branch of memory, especially when it comes to finding things. I have a good idea where the newspapers are in the morning (under the car) because I have been looking for them for years. Fortunately, I can still find my closets and I know where the chest of drawers is located. The kitchen and the living room are no problem.

Yet half my life seems to be spent searching for things. I don't want to say the objects I am trying to find have been lost or misplaced. I simply can't remember where any transient object might be. As soon as I put down a hat or a shirt in an unusual place, it becomes "lost." Half my life now seems to be spent looking for things. It often seems that Alzheimer's is making all kinds of things disappear.

This is going to be a great Christmas. I am not certain I remember where I hid all the presents. If I am going to make any sense of my life I must construct small dump sites around the house. I never realized how much disorder meant until the frustrations of Alzheimer's became mine.

It is common to have impairment of the senses in Alzheimer's disease. The ability for patients to interpret what they see, hear, taste, feel or smell declines or changes even though the sense organs may still be intact. The Alzheimer's patient should be periodically evaluated by a physician for any changes in the senses that may be correctable through glasses, dentures, hearing aids or other treatments.

Patients may also experience a

number of changes in visual abilities. For example, "visual agnosia" is a condition in which patients lose the ability to comprehend visual images. Although there is physically nothing wrong with the eyes, Alzheimer's patients may no longer be able to accurately interpret what they see due to changes in the brain. Also, their sense of perception and depth may be altered. These changes can cause safety concerns.

A loss or decrease in smell often accompanies Alzheimer's disease. Patients may experience loss of sensation or may no longer be able to interpret feelings of heat, cold or discomfort. They may also lose their sense of taste. As their judgment declines they also may place dangerous or inappropriate things in their mouths. People with Alzheimer's may have normal hearing, but they may lose the ability to accurately interpret what they hear. This may result in confusion or over-stimulation.

— *HOME SAFETY FOR*
THE ALZHEIMER'S PATIENT,
ALZHEIMER'S DISEASE
RESEARCH CENTER

———

How long is my memory? Joyce got up and

switched the television channel. I didn't no-
tice the change for five minutes when I re-
alized the story didn't seem to hang
together. I said to her, "This story doesn't
make any sense. What happened to the
guy driving the car?" I could remember but
I couldn't remember.

Ten to fifteen percent of the words I write are misspelled in crazy ways. Watching my spelling, especially when it goes out of control, is a way I keep tabs on Ol' Alzheimer's. The disease produces a literary trash pile of butchered words, once recognizable but now arranged in combinations neither I nor the spell-checker has ever seen. I have watched this syllabic exercise for months and I use it as a fingerprint of what is happening in my brain. The spawn of this destruction is growing in size and it frightens me. I may not have much time left to tinker with words. Is losing my ability to read next?

There are still a lot of children dressed as adults in politics.

When my family moved to 9th Street in Arlington, earning money after school became my foremost goal. Delivering newspapers intrigued me. There were four daily newspapers in Washington then, the *Washington Post*, the *Washington Times-Herald*, the *Evening Star*, and the *Washington Daily News*. I wasn't old enough to deliver these daily papers; boys in junior and senior high school had those routes. I broke in with shoppers, free papers delivered by youngsters, but hated the dogs that ran after me.

My first real newspaper delivery job was with the *Washington Daily News*, an afternoon tabloid with no weekend editions. Each subscriber paid weekly, and then I paid the company. With twenty customers scattered up to half a mile away, I rode my bike to shorten delivery time.

I delivered the *Evening Star* for a while, but my goal was to work for the *Washington Post*, which had absorbed the *Times-Herald*. I often walked the route with the carrier in the early-morning darkness. When the regular carrier went to college, I took the large route and kept it for four years. The money I earned helped me to make a down payment on a house when I was in high school. My father and I bought the house to rent with the idea I might need such a dwelling later.

It is too early for farewells. It is time for

memories and celebrations.

I am losing my ability to write. I see the signs of verbal atrophy every day. Cut my legs off but don't take away my ability to think, dream, and write. It is too late to reconstruct the dreams of my youth or create a new life. I am staring a monster in the face.

Silly prejudices of history haunt us through religion.

I want to tear your heart out so you can see the blood drip in my hands; then I'll put everything back so that you will bring sensitivity to your mind and think with your heart better than with your brain.

Mom, I know what death looks like. I watched you cling to life in Eldora on that teary hospital bed, a chip of ice in your mouth, dying slowly as you gave birth to a cancerous tumor. I know now how alone and vulnerable you must have felt, even in my presence, while you waited to die. Now it is my turn to begin the wait and listen in frightened silence as my brain murders my sense and destroys my body.

If children dream of the perfect aunt, my

Nell Smith was made for the job. She worked in a large clothing store in Washington, DC, and wrote a weekly commentary for a local paper in her hometown of Newton, Iowa. We were related through Grandma DeBaggio, but tracing her genealogy was tricky. Aunt Nell's lineage was carefully outlined many times, but always had to be explained again — it was less difficult tracing our relationship to President Lincoln. Only in America could a family of northern Italian peasants worm its genealogical way close to a famous president.

Visits from Aunt Nell were rare but memorable because she brought Mary Ann and me paper tickets of Sin-Sin, tiny licorice-flavored wafers knocked out of a hole of a small cardboard container. I was never sure whether my parents approved of these little presents. There was a vibrancy about Aunt Nell that was accentuated by her often flamboyant clothes and hair color, unlike any tint in the natural world.

Eventually, Aunt Nell retired from her job as a clothing store buyer and returned to Iowa. She took a job with one of her sons and bicycled to work every day for years longer than anybody thought was possible for a woman her age. She was the first writer I knew personally, but her books were filled with otherworldly encounters and spirits.

Even in this time of failing memory, I am happy to stay closeted in my mind and bring up broken memories to paw over.

Yesterday became a test of memory early in the morning, usually my best time of day. I set off in the car to pick up Briann, my niece, who needed a ride to the airport.

I had a little trouble picking out the way to her apartment on the map in my brain but I was confident of my ability to get there because it was familiar territory. I made all the right turns and recognized her place immediately. A taxi was in front of her apartment and I pulled up behind him while a young woman got in and the driver stowed her bags in the trunk.

I continued to wait on the silent street but after a few minutes I was overcome with anxiety and bewilderment. I was no longer certain I was at the proper place. My mind was flooded with images of another place nearby where she might be. I was uncertain whether this was the place I should be. Maybe this was where she lived last year and that is why she was not waiting for me.

I drove off to find the place she lived last year and eventually located it, but Briann wasn't there either. I was in careful confusion and nearly went home but first drove back to the first place I had been, to see if Briann was out on the steps with her bags. My mind was agitated and whirling out of control, my heart pounding.

I turned on her street again. As I got closer to her apartment I saw Briann and I was relieved and happy I had not gone home. The rest of the trip to the airport was uneventful, except for the subtle, aching sense of uncertainty that moves easily through me now. I saw my future and realized I was not going to be able to drive a car much longer. The crippling effects of Alzheimer's were closing in on me.

. . . .

I had an uncomplicated childhood affinity for railroads, especially those little electric trains puffing circles around Christmas trees. In a world of diesel, I imagined coal-fired boilers. My dreams were stoked by the size and power of the engine legitimized on a small scale by the men I saw at the annual model railroad display at Union Station in Washington, DC.

My love affair began with the first train set under the Christmas tree in the house on 14th Street and ended with a huge layout with trapdoors in the basement of the house on 9th Street. In between I became infatuated with small HO model trains, so much so I tried to build rolling stock from kits. One summer I bicycled to the hobby shop in Ballston and purchased a small model railroad coal-fired switch engine with money I earned from the paper route. It was an unpainted silver shell without electric motor, but it represented a past time of coal-fired engines and a present rich in dreams for a young boy.

My father was upset when he discovered my purchase. He told me to return the switch engine and to save my money instead of spending it on toys. I hid the piece of cast metal and told my father it had been returned. It was the first real break with him over the control of my life. In a small way, I started my own life the day I first lied to my father.

Do you get your hands dirty in your dreams?

Yesterday I learned what it was like to

have a rare and wonderful doctor. Colleen Blanchfield is a specialist in neurology and psychiatry, and Alzheimer's brought us, after several stumbles, to her special skills in healing. She called the family together for an occasion necessary and a little peculiar. It was to be a discussion of our future with Alzheimer's. The disease struck me but it was not just mine; it touched the entire family.

I learned some time ago what happens when you begin to tell family members about the diagnosis. My sister and cousins began to worry, however tentatively, that they, too, might be in line for a visit from Ol' Mr. Alzheimer's. Their antennae began to twitch even though we were nearly a continent apart.

Tammy and Francesco were waiting for Joyce and me when we arrived. As usual there was a long wait before Colleen finished an earlier patient and we got her full attention. She surprised me when she started the meeting by asking each of us what we thought we could get from such a forum. None of us were prepared for the question or had a clear idea what we were about to go through. I told her I didn't think I'd get anything out of it. She said that was okay.

We soon learned the meeting was to focus on living with someone with Alzheimer's, and the additional burdens on the family the disease brings. She quickly outlined a future in which I needed their help, a type of help for which they may not be prepared. Joyce ended up to be the person Colleen wanted to prepare. Tammy and Francesco had ancillary tasks looking after me when I visited them at the farm. Joyce had the largest burden but she was already carrying heavy emotional baggage, the deaths in the last six years of her father and mother. Her mother's death was particularly difficult and Joyce was required to spend days and nights with a woman who was difficult and demanding at best, paranoid at worst. Joyce was still trying to adjust to her parents' deaths when my Alzheimer's slapped her, a blow she accepted but it sent her reeling emotionally.

Colleen was animated, throwing her big mane of blond hair every which way. This was doctoring unlike any I had seen, healing and probing at the same time. Without describing the details, she was preparing us for the pain and bewilderment that lie ahead.

The meeting came to an end with Colleen asking Joyce to write down her priorities. It was then I realized how important it is to prepare not only yourself, but those around you, and how useful it is to have a wise earth mother goddess to help.

Details slather off and are tucked away in the dark litter of Alzheimer's.

On warm spring evenings my family and I sat on the back porch eating dinner. We listened to the high-pitched singing of thousands of little frogs called peepers. This serenade took place every day and night and it was not for human ears alone; it was a carefully orchestrated mating ritual devised by nature. The sound of the peepers was so continuous and enveloping that I imagined I was breathing their song.

The fallow field, often flooded by a creek running through it, was opposite the Washington and Old Dominion Railroad work station. A grassy field ran up a hill topped by a stately white house. The marshy meadow was used, with and without peepers, as a home for somnolent cows. My friends and I spent wet, dirty after-school hours collecting tiny peeper eggs with their gelatinous outer coating and a dark black center full of waiting life. I scooped them up into jars along with the dirty water. I took these jars home and watched the little peeps hatch with the care and wonder of a scientist.

There was a time, not long ago, when I seriously considered throwing all my books away. They became a reminder of my failure as a writer. Fortunately, they were rescued by Joyce, who put up cabinets for the books on the walls in a spare room. Now, with death in sight, I find it comforting to go into the room with books on the walls and pick up a book by Samuel Beckett or some other wise man of words and sorrow, and commiserate with the world. It is my way of preparing for death.

I used to sit while my brain entertained me. Ideas flew about and stories formed and laughter remained. A large array of the past and present were combined to create follies that kept me happy for hours. Now the show is over, hardly a bard exists in my memory.

This book describes an ancient time in the twentieth century.

My father had a closely trimmed mustache above his upper lip. It resembled the mustache of his father. As the two men aged, their black mustaches gradually whitened and became smaller and smaller.

I have varied slightly the steps in the cultivation of facial hair. Instead of a mustache I began with a beard. This was no ordinary beard but a statement of freedom and independence. It was a flamboyant black beard with a wide mustache that curls on its ends. As with both my father and grandfather, age manicured my facial hair until today I have a fuzzy upper lip with thick gray hairs. I have come to accept the color gray in my hair and on my face but I have not yet come to embrace its meaning.

My son, Francesco, has followed the hair-growing tradition with a flair of his own. Instead of cultivating upper-lip hair, he favored working with his scalp. He has a beautiful head of black hair falling below his shoulders when it is not tied into a ponytail. It appears he, too, is following the family tradition. When Joyce and I visited him five years ago when he lived in California, his hair hung below his waist.

It is through the growth and distribution of hair that our clan measures time.

It was an archaic time, the fifties, full of

trembling, confusion, and misunderstandings. It was also the time during which I discovered the complexity of my body and began to look at girls in a new and secret way.

In those days junior high school was more than a hiatus between grammar school and high school. It was the first step into adulthood. Growing out of elementary school was a large achievement in small lives and it made my friends and me proud to be there. Growing old, even in those young days, had a scent of hope and regret that made stomachs unsettled every day.

Swanson Junior High School was more complicated than any place I had been. It was large and there were two floors of classrooms. There was a cafeteria in which to eat lunch, and a large gym. It encompassed a time and place of hesitancy, when dancing with girls was desired and reviled at the same time.

Instead of staying in a single room students moved from room to room, studying diverse subjects with different teachers. There were books for each class and homework meant more than memorizing spelling words for a Friday test. Students were no longer treated as children, although most still acted that way.

The first day at the new school was hellish and full of hazing. On the way to and from Swanson during the first week, seventh grade students, boys and girls, were chased by older students who carried tubes of lipstick that was smeared on the faces of the new pupils.

It was easier to avoid getting smeared with red lipstick in the morning when students didn't arrive the same time. When school let out, everybody left at the same time and the older students were waiting with lipstick. I got smeared several times. We learned to run as fast as we could to avoid the older kids. As far as I could see, the hazing was condoned, to some extent, by the faculty and principal. It lasted about a week before normalcy returned.

In the time of my life, I have lived between poetry and prose, revolution and middle-class suffrage.

There are times now of light confusion when the mind lags. I have discovered the search for reality allows my instincts to take over with a quick resolution. My new motto? Let instinct rule when in doubt, with or without Alzheimer's.

★ ★ ★

Help me. Help me. Please help me. Please.

I am burdened with a "dyslectic" alphabet because I have to share my brain with Alzheimer's. I am embarrassed to tell this story because Miss Murphy taught me to be a fast, accurate typist forty-five years ago and I have retained those skills. This is not something between me and the keyboard; it is the intervention of illness.

As I type, my fingers hit unexpected keys and make words with similar sounds or rearrange letters. It began with small words. Recently I discovered the word "will" when I thought I had written "still." Another time the word "ride" turned into "rice." The word "ride" has also turned up when I intended "right," and "save" was substituted for "say." I have also noticed that the letter "B" is often substituted for the letter "P." As I wrote this my fingers struck an "M" when I was thinking "B." Sometimes this "dyslectic" alphabet goes unnoticed by me for several readings. Eye, hand, mind, the connections are weakening. Typos tell the story of the march of Alzheimer's.

There was wide diversity in the choice of

228

classes to take in junior high school, unlike the grade schools I attended. Of the electives, my father thought I should take business and typing. Neither one interested me as they sounded boring.

I realized my mistake the first day Miss Murphy walked into typing class. She was young, trim, and wore high-heeled shoes. Darkly beautiful, she was shaped like a goddess, a woman who inspired me to lust before I knew what it was. She was a recent college graduate, maybe ten years older than her students. When she walked around the room her perfume started an erotic landslide. Those times she bent over my desk to help lit me up in secret places inside. I sighed deeply when she turned her back to the class and exorcised the chalkboard. She made my heart beat faster than I thought it should, and other parts of my body responded as well, although I did not yet know what to do with these feelings.

> *Metaphor is meaning.*
> *Say yes.*
> *Say yes, you fool.*
> *No, not now.*
> *Wait for the end.*
> *The end is near.*

Memory is the past stripped of power, subject to imaginative flights, and easily manipulated into an untrustworthy cabal.

I journeyed to the grocery store yesterday with a short list of three things: the most important was cat food. I located the cat food aisle easily and as I started toward the cat food my attention was diverted by a box of Brillo pads, which we also needed. This morning when I came down to feed the cats I saw there were plenty of cat food cans and I realized I had not been the one who purchased them. It took almost twenty-four hours for me to remember the cat food I forgot to buy. My mind substituted Brillo for the cat food and erased my memory. I have vowed to write a proper list when I shop and never rely on my memory again.

Alzheimer's is hell-bent on destroying poetry and life.

I received letters of condolence from friends and strangers after I announced the Alzheimer's diagnosis. Many of the cards and letters mention Joyce and Francesco but the focus has been on me.

Joyce and Francesco suffer too, albeit in

a different way. They must watch me as I lose my mind little by little, an excruciating torture for them as well as me. What future I have is finite and marginal, marked by the catastrophe of a disease as yet incurable. It is to them I must look for comfort and help. It is to them I tell the raw stories that confirm the diagnosis and drive the dagger of sadness deeper into their chests. They are the ones battered by worry about the future, their future without me. Joyce will have memory and loneliness to replace me. Francesco will have a life circumscribed by fear he may carry the Alzheimer's gene. While I have little future, and almost certain death, their futures are full of lasting uncertainties, confusion, and burning sorrow. The silence of death, the human lot in life, is soothing compared with that.

Does sleep so mimic death that it dreams our future travail?

I have no place to go now. I sit in a chair and try to capture fleeting moments of memories.

Should I go to some exotic place and live a short happy life before the bumbling and

My disease is so hard on Joyce. It is the most unfair thing about my predicament. We have waited so long and worked hard for this time of release and thoughts of retirement. To have this come now is shattering. We should have had fun earlier instead of working constantly, but there was always the problem of money. Now Joyce looks forward to sorrow and picking up my pieces. For now, we hug more and try to understand each other truly.

Alzheimer's has taught me that sometimes it is wise to look in the same place many times for the things you desire.

There is a natural tendency for children to emulate their parents and I was no different. Both my parents smoked cigarettes. As I reached high school, I realized how close to adulthood I was and yet how little like an adult. The quickest way to become more like an adult was to smoke. I couldn't legally buy tobacco products and stealing didn't cross my mind. I looked to my world to see how close I might come to my goal.

When I was not at home, I was either at school or down the wooded bank behind the house. At the bottom of the hill were the Old Dominion railroad tracks and a narrow, quick-running creek that flowed through a county park. It was in the tangle of brush alongside the track I found what was needed for a rustic, young try at sophistication, dried sticks and hollow centers standing among the tangle of brush. Cut into the proper length, these sticks made good imitation cigarettes. With the strike of a match, I lit up and accepted my new, if hidden, refinement.

Each puff made me cough. It was a terrible experience that gave me pause, but I continued to practice clandestine sophistication. After a while, I acquired a pipe and some tobacco. My grandfather smoked a pipe with a sweet aroma and so did the boy who sat in front of me in English class, but I got no pleasure from smoking and one day threw the pipe away and forgot where the tobacco was hidden.

I go fishing because it is the only way society allows me to be a kid again, and it allows me to have time with my son.

After many years spent in the sunburnt outdoors, I now view the world through a glass window and scurry to my memory for succor. But there is not much left where dandelions once hummed of spring.

If my friends thought about it, instead of becoming emotional about me and this brain disease I have, they might see Alzheimer's as I do. It is a liberating event, freeing me to float through life and stand on its head.

The diagnosis, with little or no workable therapies to stop it, was a sentence of death as surely as birth, but more immediate.

I am running after thoughts all day. Ideas evaporate like snowflakes on a hot tin roof. A few years ago I felt normal and was as sharp mentally as my thirty-five-year-old son, Francesco. Now I can't remember his age or do the math in my head to figure it out. My mind is starting to break down. I have to wait like a hunter to capture a thought; it is tough work all day but it often flits away before I can put it on paper.

I want to cry and I do, but it is a peculiar sound, like a man choking to death. I want to scream but it won't come. Where did my voice go?

As I sit in the waiting room for the doctor, I

realize I am here at the edge of failure and of hope.

I have grown plants, herbs, and vegetables mostly, since I was six and for the last twenty-five years commercially. As a job, this activity allowed me a close look at the life and death of other species. My prolonged contact with plant life has provided me with insight on the similar life and death of my own. We scream louder.

. . . .

It was always accepted that I was college bound. Washington-Lee High School was the stop before I went away to school. This new, more serious school was much larger than Swanson and it, too, had classrooms on two floors. There were home rooms where attendance was checked and the Bible read before the academic day began. I always considered this an affliction and managed to avoid it throughout elementary and middle school. I never read the Bible and as far as I knew my family had one but I never saw anyone read it. I assumed other Catholic homes were the same way. Somehow I always managed either to be sick or to forget my Bible (Catholics have their own Bible and are taught they must not read the

Protestant version) and so I never had to read it before the class. I let others have that pleasure.

Things worked much as they had at Swanson; every forty-five minutes a bell rang for the next class. Lunch was different. The cafeteria was larger and there was smoking by students outside. Many students drove to school in their own cars, although not as many as today.

I was studious, at least in the early years, but as I got older the science, math, history, government, and even gym, began to sour. By my senior year, I began to focus on words as my future. I enrolled in a class devoted to creative writing.

The students in the class were challenged to write poetry and short stories. I managed to win a poetry award in a contest with other high school students in the Washington area.

At this point, the disease has spared my earliest memories, allowing me to dwell in another time and place from the tortures of today. My earliest memories: undershirted men after supper throwing horseshoes. Crying in a crib. Boiling water spilling on my back, leaving me scarred. These are the minutiae of my life, but I know I will have to give them up before long.

This evil disease sleeps on the edge of my consciousness, always there to remind me of its wicked strength over me.

Although nobody wanted to know the news about my Alzheimer's, friends felt slighted if someone else told them before I did.

I have been hitting the "tab" key on this computer a lot today, and before it, on other computers and many typewriters for over forty years. I do it to indent the first line of a paragraph. When I did it a few minutes ago, it was as if I had never seen a keyboard. I didn't have a clue how to do it. I looked at the keyboard for almost two minutes to remember how to indent a paragraph. If I look in a mirror, when will I no longer recognize my face?

Yet somehow, religion was important in my house. My father knew the parish priest well and for a long time he was an usher. We were invited to fish on Chesapeake Bay with Father Beatty on his large motorboat. I was too young to appreciate fishing but I understood it was good to have a priest on your side.

As a youngster, I was fascinated and proud to see my father as an usher. At a certain time every Sunday, he left the pew in which we were seated and walked up to the front of the church with a long-handled brown wicker basket. He used the basket to collect offerings. He stopped at each row of pews, passing the long-handled basket in front of each parishioner who dropped money into it.

At age sixteen, I obtained my driver's license, gave up churchgoing entirely, and became an atheist. I managed this surreptitiously. I left the house later in the morning, after my parents returned from church, telling them I was going to a later service but never went close to a church. Instead, I drove around in the car. Eventually I dropped the subterfuge and took the heat. There was a big blowup with lots of anger and loud words. It could have been worse but my parents, to my surprise, were realists and sadly accepted my behavior. I was thankful, but I remained on the course I set for myself.

Why am I possessed with the longing to have a grandchild? Let those angry genes that put me here die with me.

The interviews with Noah Adams on public radio sprang from the same nexus as this book. It was a way to talk to people about a troubling disease that affects millions of Americans, yet is little understood by the public. I have known Noah and his wife, Nina, for years. We have a common interest in the rich earth of gardens and in fresh food produced in backyards. I broached the idea to Noah in a telephone conversation one afternoon. He told me he had the same idea when he read of my condition, but he thought it unseemly to push the idea on me.

The interview came together at our farm in Loudoun County, Virginia. I had undergone interviews like this before, but Joyce and Francesco had not. They were nervous and uncertain. What would they say with meaning and relevance? I tried to reassure them not to worry; the questions Noah asked would release their inner thoughts.

Noah arrived with a soundman and a producer and a modest amount of equipment. Before the interview began, we chatted in Francesco and Tammy's living room in front of a crackling fire. Noah held a microphone in his hand and began talking to us casually, steadying those with uneasiness. He talked about everything but

Alzheimer's. He exposed his Ohio boyhood and his first radio job failure. He looked at the soundman, perched next to me, and said casually, "Is everything ready?" He nodded and we were off. The interview took over an hour but with skill and sensitivity Noah and his producer found the essence of what we had to say in about twelve minutes of tape.

My intention in both this book and the radio interviews is to break through the sense of shame and silence Alzheimer's has engendered. I want people with the disease to come forward, unafraid of exposing their illness, and tell the world what it is like. Doctors and advocates can help, but there is nothing like personal stories to humanize the silent, destructive power of this illness. The more we talk about it and expose Alzheimer's, the greater the chance a cure will be found quickly.

The best thing that happened to me in high school was getting a job on the *Northern Virginia Sun* when I was in eleventh grade. The *Sun*, a small daily paper then in Arlington, was saved from deserved obscurity by a group of important Democrats, including Clayton Fritchy, the publisher. I was one of several students who worked for the teen-page editor, a no-nonsense woman who put together a daily page about schools largely written by teen-agers.

I was happy in ways I had never experienced. I was, for the first time, being paid for writing, twenty-five cents an inch of printed copy. At the end of every month, I spread all the squibs and stories I had written, counted the inches, and submitted a bill to the newspaper. I scribbled so many stories the editor of the page hired me to work after school. It was here I fell in love with journalism and got a small taste of the power a writer has and the backlash that can come from it.

With no camera and little money, I went to a part of Arlington called Rosslyn, a seedy district filled with pawnshops and rooms to let above them. I purchased a cheap camera in a pawnshop to record the action for my first big story, an exposé of hazing practices by high school fraternities and sororities, outlawed by the state, but still in business. It involved things of which students were aware but the general public was not. I wrote a story, including photographs of fraternity brothers using huge paddles on the backsides of plebes.

The story was a sensation but it did not

endear me to the school principal, a small, angular man who ordered me out of class and into his office. He wanted an explanation. This was the first time something like this happened to me and I was scared but defiant. I told the principal I was covering the news at the school. If he didn't like what I uncovered, he should change what was happening at the school, not pillory the reporter. The idealism of youth prevailed.

After I reached forty, I cast aside youthful energy and dreams and hugged an uneventful life. This muted life left me blind to my hungry past, emotionless but trailing hurried whispers.

It may appear to be just another illness, especially of the elderly, but Alzheimer's is a unique and wrenching disease that destroys the mind, without which you lose your sense of being human. In its early stages, when you are most sensitively aware, you watch helplessly as you slowly lose yourself. Memory disappears. Language is gone. You forget who you are and become lost and dependent. Yet you continue on in silence, the body unsure and hesitating, as the diabolical disease proceeds to kill you slowly by destroying what remains of your body and your life. But the destruction continues, doing its best to uproot your loved ones and dip their hearts in the fire.

My mind is becoming one-dimensional. I have almost lost my ability to hold two thoughts simultaneously. Along with this is the long, frustrating wait for the word I need in conversation.

When my doctor prescribed one-half hour of reading each day, I was charmed and bewildered. That something so simple as reading affects the brain made immediate sense. She wasn't kidding. She wanted me to work my brain, play its keys, and search its private places. It was a return to an earlier time when words encircled my small world and hope was a genie without a bottle.

This brain exercise wouldn't be a cure but it might slow its passage toward atrophy. Talking and reading were how I got started filling my brain after birth. Now I was asked again to work my brain, this time to keep me alive a little bit longer.

The world in which I grew, long gone now, was made serene for me by those who worked hard to love me. That happy private world has disappeared and the only things of that time to remain are memories, and now they slip away. Love can help stabilize my unsteady life, but even it lacks the power to restore my spirit and return me to the happy world as it was before Alzheimer's darkened my sight and roiled my soul.

Joyce gave me a beautiful set of CDs this Christmas featuring jazz of the past, the time of my youth and earlier. I was delighted and eagerly picked a disc. This was new technology with which I was unfamiliar. We called Francesco to find out which side of the disc was up. I felt very old that day, older than I have ever felt in my life.

One Halloween night, teenagers, many of whom I knew from high school classes, rampaged through Westover, a small wayside shopping strip surrounded by brick apartments a few blocks from where I once lived on 14th Street. These teenagers, from middle- and upper-class families, ran amok breaking store and car windows, and flattening auto tires in a darkness they thought protected them. They swirled through the streets yelling obscenities and owning the night.

There were many bright students I knew in the group. It took the quiet, sedate community by surprise, leaving parents and county officials breathless, befuddled, and worried. It was an event its participants could not fully explain, an explosion of undirected youthful energy exploding in a wicked show of group dynamics.

Many participants in what was labeled a riot were called before juvenile judges at the courthouse. What was happening in the shadows of world wars as America muscled its way to world power and small towns emptied to fill cities in a catastrophic embrace?

Something has been lacking in these words I have scribbled. It is the life around me in the members of my family. They are wary of losing their privacy in the onslaught of my words and careful to hide their sorrow from the world. This is a very private thing I have put on display, a show of nakedness unusual for a man and difficult for his family. They are hesitant to put their thoughts in words the world will read, a method of self-exposure with which they are unfamiliar and wary. I continue to urge them to take notes of their thoughts and feelings. In the meantime, I write what I observe of them and provide them with the ability to amend my words.

My high school days were suspended in a time of hope and evil. The beginning of the end of government-ordered racial separation began with a U.S. Supreme Court decision. In Arlington there was no greater evil, at the time, than George Lincoln Rockwell's American Nazi Party. Rockwell took residence in the county with the help of several prominent people, including at least one person on the county board and a school board member. There was also an active organization promoting the idea of sending black Americans back to Africa.

Integration was the overarching topic bedeviling Virginia, and the nation. Some Virginia school systems closed public schools, and new private all-white schools blossomed, leaving black children without education. Arlington County was considerably more liberal than most parts of Virginia and schools stayed open. At W-L and other schools, there was tension in the air. Some students formed a Nazi party secretly meeting in school. Outside school, a wariness was palpable.

Local efforts in Arlington began to

smooth the way to a transition to integrated schools. One of the first was an interracial dinner including high school students. I was one of the participants. It was an evening set up to test whether the state would stop "race mixing," as it was called by segregationists. The dinner was held in a large hall at the Unitarian Church in Arlington.

Reporters representing newspapers and television stations all over the country were present. Everybody was on edge, except perhaps the students selected from all the schools in the county. My colleagues and I ate dinner, chatted among ourselves, and answered questions asked by the reporters as we filed out. There had been no attempt to stop the event.

Shirley Elder, the *Sun* reporter assigned to the event, came to me and asked me to write the story of the event for the next day's paper. I was elated and went back to the empty newsroom and struggled with words for an hour or more. I confronted what all journalists bump against when an event is without explosive drama, but is historic at the same time. The next day my story was on the front page as I had written it.

★ ★ ★

Joyce is a sensitive woman with an artistic gift of color and form. She studied long and worked hard. No one could have prepared for the struggle I have presented her. In the wake of the death of her parents over the last decade, I slapped her with a large emotional hurdle, my slow, wretched death by Alzheimer's.

I cannot know her pain except as she has allowed me to see it. She does not come from a family of volubility and openness but thirty-seven years of marriage during which I withheld none of my pain and hunger may have changed her.

It is not easy to expose what has been secret or unsaid. In a place like America where emotion is often denied and strength is measured by how much is withheld, it is much more difficult to shed tears in words for the world to read. My story is also her story in many ways and her story is mine. Each of our stories may cover the same terrain but they will be indulged and viewed from different points of view. Even the way the world thinks about our roles differs; she is the suffering wife, I am the dying husband.

I hope we can throw the storyline away, strip the protective cover, and tell how we hurt individually from this small, private human catastrophe.

Joyce seemed to absorb the bad news of my illness and life went on with little change. As always when the holidays approached, she took a leave of absence from her studio. Before long, however, her sense of organization eroded. Things she began were all left lying. Every once in a while her former self peeked from beneath her shrouded face.

Then she began staying up later at night; sometimes all night. She has always been a late riser and she pokes fun at my early-to-bed habit, but there were days when she was still in bed at 2 p.m. I rationalized the change — she went to bed at 7 a.m. and she was deserving of seven hours' sleep.

Slowly motivation became almost nonexistent. She spent hours reading the newspapers and watching television, and then berated herself for getting nothing accomplished. She wanted to take time from her studio at the Torpedo Factory Art Center in Alexandria to paint the bedroom. All we managed was ordering new furniture for the bedroom. She wanted to help me have time to write and make my life easier, but she wasn't dressed in time to make dinner. That, too, continued the self-deprecation.

It made me cry to watch her struggle with the silent demons of her depression.

Finally she sought medical help and after a few tries with different drugs, her depression began to abate and her smile returned. She accepts surprise with a grin now.

Going to college was something my parents had done and it was expected of me too. I didn't care where I went as long as it was far away from home. I settled on the University of Arizona, nearly a continent away.

I got on the airplane and flew to Tucson clutching my bible, J. D. Salinger's *Catcher in the Rye*. This best-seller about youths in New York opened my eyes about the world and its ways. Almost the minute the plane landed, I began looking for "phonies" and easily spotted them tangled in their insecurities.

Inside the terminal I spotted two boys my age and walked over and introduced myself. They were waiting for the bus to the university. Both of them were New Yorkers. Finally, the three of us hired a taxi and were delivered to the campus.

The campus was a new world, filled with tall, upright buildings. The Arizona heat was another surprise. Cars parked on campus, many of them new, were covered with parachute cloth to protect the finish from the brutal sun. The earth was a dry inferno and it made me sweat less. I stood on the sidewalk and looked at the building soon to become my domicile, and wanted to go home. The hot, dry sun saved me from showing my tears.

In those days the United States was inching its way into Vietnam and protests were beginning. ROTC was mandatory at the university and I simply boycotted it. In class and in the cafeteria I continued to mentally identify phonies.

Before long I was skipping classes. My final fling was a day spent wandering with Bob Hurwitt, one of the chums I met that first day at the airport. We filled backpacks with food and wine and hitched a ride to the rough, hard mountains outside Tucson. The cheese melted and the sharp stones made our sneakers almost useless.

The idea was to walk back to school by a scenic route. As night fell, Bob and I were high among the rocks in an unfamiliar sharp wilderness. In the distance a light winked and we stumbled toward it. Approaching a brightly lit ranch we were greeted by an angry man with an ugly carbine. He thought we were chicken thieves.

He pointed the way back to the highway and Bob and I began a long trek down the driveway filled with sharp, high, dry grass. Under the light of a bright moon, we passed a car parked along the side of the drive, windows fogged with passion. We walked a long time before car lights illuminated our backs. The couple, students at the university, picked us up and we returned to campus.

Within a few days I climbed on a cross-country Greyhound headed for home. Bob and I found a common bond in words and literature, a link that has kept our friendship alive to this day, even though we dwell on opposite coasts.

I awake in the dark morning without awareness of what day of the week it is. I wait for the newspaper or the radio to locate me in time. The day of the week, the hour of the day has little meaning for me even when I remember. I float in my own chaotic world, grateful to know I am still alive.

There are moments when I no longer remember routine chores, but my mind has not lost all my familiar motions.

I make an effort and suddenly what I

could not remember begins to take shape in fits and starts. Memory comes to my rescue.

It has been several months since I made a bank deposit, a chore I accomplished with ease as recently as June, and it is only January. Thinking about the process, trying to resurrect the memory of how this simple task is done with paper and pen, eluded me. Flashes of anger and frustration exploded in my head. I remembered clearly having done the familiar business chore but I was now having trouble understanding it.

It wasn't until I held the deposit slip in my hand and felt my familiar pen that I began to slowly unravel the mystery of this once-simple task. The struggle to bring meaning out of inanimate objects and to remember simple, familiar tasks is now on another level.

Throughout our lives we control nature's human urges — anger, slothfulness, murder, revenge, wars, all the dangers that trouble our societies. We honor life in the face of certain death. In our own familiarity, we seek grandeur and strength. Yet there is no real nobility in the face of death whether it comes with a startle or a grimace. It is always a dirty mess. The reason we erect stone markers to the dead is to remind us of our frailty and animal cunning. Sleep, sweet beast.

Without college to protect me, I had to find a job and landed at *U.S. News and World Report*, then under the control of David Lawrence, an aging shepherd of the right wing. Mike Boggs, then a copyboy and friend from high school, helped me get the job. Pay was meager, $40 a week, and I was paid in cash stuffed in a little yellow envelope. I lived at home and needed little, so I threw the unopened pay envelopes in the bottom drawer of the dresser.

Copyboys ran errands around the big newsroom and the offices surrounding it. There were usually at least two copyboys and we performed an hourly run, shuffling paper back and forth among offices. There was always a lot of time off and we read books and chatted politics. It was in the days just before and after Fidel Castro overthrew the dictatorship in Cuba and there was a lot of talk about it. One morning Mike and I discussed a Fair Play for Cuba Committee advertisement in the *New York Times*. The woman who shuffled paperwork to copyboys overheard the conversation.

"Don't get involved with those commies," she warned. "You'll never get another job. Somebody in the FBI will have a membership list within a week."

I bicycled to work and wore pants so old the front pockets were gone. Lunch was spread on the nearby grass green park with the young women who worked in the business office on the first floor. I was eighteen, legal drinking age then, and for a while I kept a bottle of Chianti in the copyboy's desk to prove my manhood and to refresh the bag lunch my mother made.

Once a week, as production night drew near, I stayed late. It was a long day but I got dinner free across the street at the company cafeteria. When Mike left to go to school in Mexico, I became head copyboy and had to stay after midnight. On those nights I was allowed to take a cab home at company expense.

I enjoyed the copy editors. They sat in a big circle in the middle of the room editing the news stories, written by rewrite men, a few correspondents, and editors in offices that wrapped the edge of the room. Each of these grizzled editors was a "pop-out" individualist. The head of the copydesk, a middle-aged man, threw paper clips at women's behinds all day long. Another copy editor chewed paper clips; another hummed continuously. The guy who sat closest to the copyboys flipped pencils into the air and caught them without looking while reading copy.

My mind is so fertile and alive this morning I am almost afraid to take my three-mile walk. If I am caught in the midst of a lovely brainstorm of words and ideas, I may be unable to catch the idea or thought before it disappears. I postponed my walk to better enjoy the explosions of words awakening my brain on this bright winter morning.

I am more aware of the world now, the tiny insignificant things especially. I am beginning to be more childlike. For an artist this may have some advantages. As a fifty-eight-year-old man it has many drawbacks. I am losing precious memory and complex ideas become twisted. I am becoming a child again against my will.

I am so sick of hearing about technology I can't wait to lose my mind. Technology is nothing without humanity and we will lose everything if we forget that.

Noah Adams of National Public Radio sent me mail from his offices after the first broadcast of the family interview. There were two letters with interesting stories from individuals with experience of Alzheimer's.

Pamela Stewart, of Oxford, Iowa, lost her husband to Alzheimer's and remembered it in a poem to me. Her husband died two years ago, she wrote, ten years after onset.

"I wrote a lot of poetry during that time," she recounted. "It helped me and I have shared some of the poems with friends who are dealing with the same problem. Hence the poem which took shape in my mind as I listened and committed to paper when I got home."

ALZHEIMER'S REVISITED

Today I heard the voice of
a 58-year-old man,
as he spoke of losing his memory,
word by word, thought by thought.
He said, "The only thing I never forget
is that I have Alzheimer's disease."

As he spoke of exercising his mind,
I pictured, once again, my husband

sitting at his desk, writing his name,
over and over, letters missing,
writing fading into a meaningless scrawl.
Then a group of near-perfect signatures.
Strong will and determination to not let go,
beaten by the inevitable progress
of a mind-stealing illness.

At that moment I wanted to reach out
and tell this family that I too could
never forget that I loved one
who had Alzheimer's disease.
I wanted to tell them, too,
that times of pure love and closeness
will be theirs to savor and enjoy.

The simple accomplishments
are like a mountain climbed.
A victory against all odds.
That the act of unlearning
is like a book read backwards.
The words and stories there
to be unscrambled, interpreted,
and imprinted on the minds of others.

Another letter, from a woman in Issaquah, Washington, told a story of a friend:

FROM WHAT I HAVE OBSERVED of the disease, each person is affected differently, so I do not intend to generalize from what happened to my elderly friend Emily, but with her, when the words and memories dropped away, her essence became more pronounced and delightful . . .

Because Alzheimer's became too difficult to deal with, her husband finally placed her in a small nursing home in 1983. The time of adjustment was difficult, but once she felt secure in the routine of the home, her intelligence and caring continued to manifest itself, even though she was in her late 80's and had no memory to speak of.

One of the funniest episodes I remember was the time I picked up books from a small distribution company whose location was on the hillside above the nursing home. The owner was laughing about something he saw that morning — a little old lady in a pink dress was making her way craftily across the flat roof of the nursing home, when suddenly a white-coated orderly threw open the door to the roof and ran frantically after her.

When I finished my business at the distribution company, I stopped at the nursing home. "Sharon," I said to the head nurse, "I hear you had a patient on the roof."

Startled, she said, "Don't tell Mr. Braman." And I realized the little old lady in pink was my friend Emily who had seen a workman go up on the roof the day before and *remembered* and calculated the route to the freedom she loved more than just about anything.

. . . .

By the time I reached twenty, I was tough to love as a son. I had given up Catholicism, one of the pillars of my father's life. I had forgone college, one of the keys to getting ahead in life for my parents. When I had a job it was humble, and with little redeeming social value. Could the kid be saved? So what does the old man do? He takes the whole family on a grand tour of Europe, from Italy to France with stops in Switzerland and Austria.

We saw all the sights in Paris. I wandered alone in the deserted market district where the air was the color of granite with a feeling of empty fear in the air. The biggest surprise was watching my puritanical father at one of those tourist-trap girlie shows with nearly nude women kicking up a storm on stage.

In Switzerland everything was so orderly

it made you want to spit on the street. Every man carried a briefcase and the hotel pulled down the cover at night and put a wrapped chocolate in the exact place where your head was to lie.

It was Italy for which my family had been waiting. Watching the men in their tight clothing saunter down the street with jackets hanging over the shoulders was to see slow-moving sophistication. The women had an attitude to match the men, strong, earthy, and openly sexual.

Motorbikes, bicycles, and cars clogged the polluted streets and alleys of Rome. Dark shadows of shade protected us from the hot sun and there were dainty chairs on which to sit while sipping a drink.

From Rome the family darted to Venice, floated on the canals, walked over the bridges, peeked in the churches without chairs, and watched the artisans heating metal and hammering it smooth and shapely. For all the sightseeing, there was one event more important than others, the car trip to Romans, the village of my Grandpa DeBaggio's birth.

Romans was a dirt road kind of place where doorways hung with bright, beaded cord. We stopped at the church first to inspect the register of births. We counted the

Di Biasio's, as the name had been before the transatlantic separation, centuries ago. By the time we finished the tour in the church's birth records, the whole village knew Americans were there. A man waited for us when we returned to the street. He was wearing the local wooden shoe and spoke English, a version of which he learned in Texas and Iowa.

My father wanted to meet any relatives who might still be there and we were taken to see an old man who stood at proud attention in front of his small detached house and spoke Friulani in response to our English. Then we went to a cramped little house with an earthen floor and a hole in the roof for a chimney. This, we were told, was Grandpa's home in Italy before he was lost to America.

The scourge of my young life, especially in school, was the Bible reading that was required every morning. How this practice got started I don't know, but it was routine in public schools I attended in Virginia. Somehow I managed to avoid uttering a Bible passage throughout my ten years in public schools, through either luck or illness. It was not just the idea of standing up in front of the class that weakened my knees; that was bad enough. Reading words that seemed to be in a language almost like English but not quite recognizable really made me nervous. My shyness was a huge deterrent when it came to standing up in front of the class for any reason.

I was brought up in a Catholic family in a place with few Catholics. To my parents, being a Catholic was serious, but reading the Bible was not something I ever saw them do. It was the Mass on Sunday, not the Bible, to which my parents clung.

In the background lurked a remote but palpable fear that we might be rounded up any day and killed for our religion. Catholics had been hanged in the South and the Klan was still active when I grew up. When the time came, later in life, to make my own choices it was easy for me to adopt an atheist position. I had enough of religious zealotry.

In school Protestant Bibles were used and I was forbidden by Catholic Church law to read such books as the King James version. I took the ban seriously because my father did. It meant that when my day to read the Bible came around I had to bring my Douay Bible to school and expose myself as a Catholic, and this I wanted to avoid; it was bad enough being teased for my skinny body and shyness.

Although I was out of school when the practice of reading the Bible in public schools finally ended, I shouted for joy just at the memory of all the fear I underwent.

Cold winter morning iced in fear,
  sidewalks lathered slick with white stuff.
Filled with images of cobbles.
My bony head, immobile, eyes closed.
Images of coffins.
Rigidity of death.
  The way it ends.
  No matter age or how hard you tried.
    Or lied.
What accomplished.
How get through this.
Same tunnel as before. Keep going,
    moving ahead.
    Alone or not.
No matter.
Yelp of pain, smile of pain.
No matter.
Secret mind talk without remembrance.
    Cobble me a cobble.
Shroud. Where is shroud?
You can't death me without shroud.

No bury; hot coals leaping, bright sparks and flesh sizzle.

Dust to dust.

Amen

— MY LAST WILL AND TESTAMENT, JANUARY 22, 2000

I got to like Mike while we worked together at *U.S. News and World Report.* Eventually, he went to Mexico to study at Mexico City College where he fell hard for his guitar and life.

During those days as a copyboy I discovered Henry Miller's work, which was still banned in the United States. His books, published in France by Olympia Press, were autobiographical, freewheeling, and sexually frank, exactly what a late-teenage boy brought up in a Catholic family needed most.

One of the copy editors at *U.S. News* had spent time in France as a wire service correspondent. He loved to talk about his adventures in Paris and other cities in France. He interviewed Picasso, among other luminaries, and told us he watched the famous artist go swimming nude. He read all of Miller's books and told me about them.

I obtained the name and address of a mail order store in Paris and ordered

Miller titles. Before long the mail brought a card addressed to me from U.S. Customs explaining the books were banned in the United States and had been seized and were scheduled to be destroyed unless I proved I had a scholarly use for them.

Unfortunately, I was not the first person in my family to read the Customs notice; my mother also had the pleasure. That night was not a pretty affair as my father grilled me about what I read and why I desired to possess banned books.

I corresponded with Mike and told him of the seizure of books from Paris. Mike told me of a bookstore in Mexico City that stocked all of Miller's books up to that point and shipped them anywhere in the world. I was hesitant about ordering them, but looked upon this as an opportunity to join Mike in Mexico City where he shared an apartment with a fellow former student from high school.

I led a sheltered middle-class life and was unprepared for what I found in Mexico City as the train crawled through the slums. There seemed to be endless miles of cardboard and scrap-wood shanties on bare ground. Children and adults openly urinated outside their leaky shacks. It was dusk as the train pulled into the station and I had the eerie feeling I was walking into a mysterious, surreal Brueghel painting.

Parents have many responsibilities, including teaching their children how to eat grapefruit.

With failing memory, it is difficult to write long passages without getting lost in words. Where does the story go? Why does the pencil tremble? I see only the structure of words, their meaning elusive. I am often able to write only a sentence or two, enough to sketch what was to be brawny and complex. Do you understand I am not dying, just disappearing before your eyes?

On an early Sunday morning in July, I waited nervously for the driveway gravel to announce my thirty-five-year-old son's arrival. Francesco is our only child and I asked him to drive me into Washington, DC. Normally I would have insisted on driving myself, but more than a year ago, I plunged into forgetfulness and memory loss. Although my dementia is young and hardly identifiable to the walking-around world, my brain has begun to abandon me, leaving insecurity, un-self-confidence, and anxiety.

Once in a great while I am treated to a transitory nocturnal hallucination of bright-yellow lights dancing on walls and ceilings.

One of the important failings that beset me was my inability to picture in my mind where places were and how to get to them. I can still negotiate the familiar streets of Arlington, Virginia, where I have lived most of my fifty-eight years. Trying to find my way around the mysterious streets of the District of Columbia is more than I can manage, even with detailed instructions.

Francesco had not arrived and I was anxious. I started walking back and forth between the kitchen and the living room. I pushed the living-room drapes aside for a better look at the driveway and the street. Francesco lives on a five-acre farm in Chantilly, Virginia, with two houses and a large brick barn and as much wildlife as anybody could want. Following in his father's footsteps, he grows and sells herb and vegetable plants in greenhouses there. It is about forty minutes from the Arlington house. What if he overslept or got stuck in traffic?

I started a backyard farm with my wife, Joyce, nearly thirty years ago after I gave up journalism in frustration at wimpy editors and sly newspaper owners with monied friends who wanted front-page coverage of non-news. About the same time, Joyce struck out on her own as an artist and she still maintains a studio at the Torpedo Factory Art Center along the Potomac River in Alexandria, Virginia.

In the small backyard behind our 1918 wooden house on Ivy Street in Arlington, Virginia, I began an apprenticeship with the earth and dirty hands. After a short period of growing tomatoes and cabbages for our own desperate needs, I realized ignorantly that there was something incredible about growing food from the earth. To make a life with a tiny backyard farm, I had to know more about growing plants, particularly herbs, which were an underrated crop, plants in which I eventually specialized. I haunted the Library of Congress, searching for growing information. I also contacted academics in the horticulture field and bled them of their secrets.

Our little backyard was an unlikely place to begin farming. Next to us on 10th Street was a used-car lot and opposite it a new-car dealer. Years earlier, livery stables occupied the property opposite what is now the used-car lot. When the horses died, their bodies were buried on the property next to ours. Under the hot, dark asphalt of today's used-car lot lie bones of dead horses who provided transportation in another era.

Eventually our backyard sprouted several greenhouses and became one of the first successful urban herb farms in America. Despite the hard work and frustrations caused by nature, it was a joy to watch our little idea grow into a business that supported us and helped send Francesco to college.

As I reached my fifty-seventh birthday, I came upon the greatest challenge I ever faced. I thought I was breaking into pieces. I found it hard to concentrate because shards of memory kept disappearing suddenly. It took me by surprise and left me angry and bewildered. My initial feeling was that a steady diet of anxiety and long days were the cause. But what was responsible for my inability to remember the names of familiar plants? After a long series of tests, I was told I had Alzheimer's. Without a cure for the disease, I realized my days of 100-hour weeks were over.

At the end of spring, we closed our Arlington plant business. It ended an important part of our lives and there was happiness and tears celebrating nearly thirty years of dirty hands. We no longer had our people of the spring and fall to brighten our days, customers yearning for a connection with the past and finding it in a garden of herbs. The streets, once full of customer's cars, could now rest.

Although Joyce and I continue to live in the house on Ivy Street, we consolidated our plant-growing business in Francesco's capable hands in Chantilly, Virginia. I was free now of other duties and could devote myself to writing during what I considered my last years. I had managed to write, or collaborate with others, on three books about gardening and herbs in the last ten years while working in the greenhouse. These were fine books but not what I dreamed of writing when I was in high school, when James Joyce and Henry Miller were my idols.

For a few short weeks after the diagnosis, I thought my life was over. I didn't know where to turn. I thumbed through scientific reports trying to understand what happened to me. I didn't ask why but I wondered when the illness's intrusion began, and where it came from. Was it my father or my mother who passed the bad gene to me unknowingly? Or was it a freak occurrence?

After those weeks in silent introspection, I realized this slow-moving disease offered a great opportunity to me. The Alzheimer's diagnosis freed me at last to write seriously and well if my gift of language did not fail me.

Francesco's car crunching the front-yard gravel disturbed my thin thought at 8 a.m., more than an hour before the start of the panel discussion in which I had been asked to take part. The panel was a small part of ten days of intense discussion at the World Alzheimer's Congress.

I took one last look in the bathroom mirror and combed my hair again. My head was quickly filling with white hair but enough dark strands remained for me to remember the lustrous black that crowned my youthful head. This falling, long face and that nearly white mustache was what I feared all my life — my father's image, an old man, not even a grandpa. It wasn't as if I hadn't earned these stripes of age honestly, but I'd trade them now to be thirty-five again even with all its wonder and insecurity.

Generationally different but obviously in the mold of his father, Francesco is a young man with black hair hanging down his back, almost to his waist, and a mind as sharp as a steel trap. I fear for him now like I never had to do when he was in high school and college on his own. I see him watch me sometimes, searching for a clue whether he will end his life as I am mine, mentally crippled, bewildered, helpless, waiting for death to end my pain and panic.

We got in my beat-up, peeling Ford Explorer, Francesco at the wheel, and headed downtown. I began telling Francesco what had happened the last few days. A whirlwind had ripped through the preparation for the panel discussion. For several days it appeared I would be the only participant. No one with Alzheimer's in the Washington area except me, apparently, was willing to participate. At the last minute, Lisa Gwyther from Duke University, the panel moderator, located some willing men and women with Alzheimer's in Ohio and brought them to Washington.

A week earlier I was preparing for an interview with Madeleine Nash, a *Time* magazine medical correspondent. She planned to meet me Saturday, July 8, the day before the Alzheimer's Conference was to begin. She didn't show up for the interview and I called her at her home in Illinois. When she answered the phone, I realized *Time* had changed plans. Instead of offering the story after the convention, they decided at the last minute to have a story before the Alzheimer's Congress began. Madeleine Nash stayed home and worked the phones and wrote words.

By now Francesco was tooling through Washington streets. We were following a map given us by the Alzheimer's Association and it was taking us all over the place.

"I don't know where we are. Do you know where you are?" I asked Francesco.

"I don't think so," he said.

He did know and we got there in plenty of time, no thanks to the map.

The panel was predictable, a question-and-answer format with the moderator guiding us through the hoops. The large room was packed and silent. We all had stories to tell and Gwyther knew them and helped us tell them well. I choked when I heard one panelist's story. After going through a long battery of tests, and a time of anxious waiting, his doctor sent a letter to tell his patient he had Alzheimer's — a doctor out of the same school as the one I had in the beginning of my battle with Alzheimer's.

I am learning there are many levels of

memory. Where am I in the process of dwindling returns brought on by that deliciously foreign-sounding disease, Alzheimer's? I can still type letters with some authority, although with many typos. Some people tell me I still have more than enough speech. In the morning, I can rarely remember what clothes I wore the day before. Notes at different locations around the house remind me to take medication. The day after I write a letter, I may remember the envelope but not its content. After some thought and several minutes of struggle, and maybe some stuttering in my brain, I may sometimes remember to whom the letter was addressed.

There was a time I was under the influence of the French Surrealists and I cataloged my dreams daily. Those youthful days are gone without a firm memory. Now my dream world, when it exists at all, is absorbed before I recognize it. Last night, however, a dream awakened me with its silent disruptive power and left me limp with its frightening images. The dream's imaginative force was so great I struggled to breathe.

The dream was a black-and-white "B" movie. The main character worked in a store ringing up sales much like me, but to my horror, none of the items for sale were priced. The merchandise in the store was unfamiliar to me, so much so I didn't know how it was used. All the customers were tough and surly, constantly changing their minds and making threats.

At one point in the dream I went to the bathroom in the store, but I kept losing my way in a hall of mirrors. It was a disorderly world in which I moved, with signs upside-down and backward.

Now my dreams, those secrets of the night, betray me. I cannot hide from the mental contamination of Alzheimer's. I pulled the covers over my head to flee my growing inadequacy, fear, and failure.

When I was fully awake and I caught my breath, I realized this nightmare was just another billboard reminding me my life was no longer mine. The disease has wrested me from the command of my skills and even the secrets of sleep. Alzheimer's has followed me to the bedroom and captured my dreams. Now I am certain there is no place to hide.

Where does this dance of hope lead?

Mexico forty years ago was a kaleidoscope. Every corner brought me face-to-face with laughter and sadness. It was a startling show.

One day I saw a young boy with his pants down, his back against a building, relieving himself in the middle of the busy city with crowds of people on the streets and sidewalks.

Mike and I saw another poor kid, maybe eight or nine years old, alone in the street begging one day. We felt sorry for him and brought him home for some food and a good night's sleep. Mike spoke fluent Spanish. In the morning, we packed the child a lunch. After he left I went to the bathroom and discovered the kid's footprints on the toilet seat.

Mike's apartment was on Kant Street and I was happy to be in a place honoring philosophers. Down the street from the apartment was a lovely house with a narrow metal-gated entrance. What was seen from the street was a hint of a delightful little garden. During the entire month I was there, two men worked on the gate. Each day they sanded the rust from the metal to prepare it for painting. Every night the damp air created more rust. The offspring of those two workmen may now be sanding the gate for the next generation of the family that lives there.

Alzheimer's remains a poorly understood disease, but one study suggests a possible link between it and early life.

One of the University of Washington researchers involved in the study, Dr. Victoria M. Moceri, an epidemiologist who presented the research in the journal *Neurology*, said she was not claiming she had found the cause of the debilitating illness.

"There are many different causes of Alzheimer's disease," Dr. Moceri said. "One factor will not be unique to every person. There are genetic risk factors."

Aware that early childhood factors play roles in a wide variety of other illnesses, like cardiovascular disease, the researchers reasoned that the same might be true for Alzheimer's. They were especially interested because the areas of the brain showing the first signs of the disease take the longest to develop, often maturing well into adolescence, as crucial synaptic and other connections are made.

So they studied 700 members of a Washington H.M.O. who were 60 or over. Of those, 393 had Alzheimer's, and the rest showed no signs of dementia.

The researchers say they found a link between the patients with Alzheimer's and the conditions of their childhood homes. For example, those with more than five siblings, which the researchers associated with lower income generally, at least when the subjects were children, had 39 percent more cases of Alzheimer's than other members of the group. Those who grew up in the suburbs, on the other hand, were less likely to develop the illness than those who grew up in poorer farm areas or more crowded cities, places where children would be more likely to be exposed to infectious diseases.

— *THE NEW YORK TIMES*,
FEBRUARY 1, 2000

Something happened last night so frightening I hesitated to write about it. Now I want to write about it but my memory got lost yesterday.

Joyce came across a pot I made thirty years ago. I built it from unamended fire clay to which I added small particles in green pigment. It was then given a clear glaze. It made a sturdy, medium-sized pot with a faded green-grass color punctuated with tiny bursts of dark-green dribbles in an irregular pattern throughout. I recognized the decrepit pot, but I had no immediate memory of making it.

It took almost twenty-four hours for me to dredge up this little story from my memory. I now live for encounters with the past like this. It is a way of proving to myself I am not ready yet for the trash can. Small things matter so much when the uncomfortable end is in sight.

Time moved slowly in Mexico, so slowly I was no longer certain in which century I lived. I spoke no Spanish and it was the first time I was without language.

Men and women clung to the sides of buses for free rides. Women inside the bus openly breast-fed their babies without any sense of embarrassment.

It was good to know, in a city as vibrant as Mexico City, there were books in English by Henry Miller for sale. I found the store easily and bought a copy of every Henry Miller they stocked. Later, when I returned and crossed the border on the way back home, an American customs official asked me to open my bag for inspection. I had carelessly placed a Miller book I was reading at the top of the bag. The customs officer immediately took the book and asked me to dump the contents of the bag on the counter. He seized three more Miller books. The woman behind me saw what happened and in a bewildered voice said to me, "Why did they take your books away?" I told her they were banned in the United States, something she had never heard. That was the way of life then; police had the power to control what you read.

After many years spent in the sunburnt outdoors, I now view the world through a glass window and scurry to my memory for comfort. But there is not much left where dandelions once hummed of spring.

Is life real when we do not comprehend our surroundings or recognize a heartbeat?

There is always something lurking around the corner. For me it is a life without a life. A world of silence and confusion. The scent of nursing homes and tears. A stumbling life of humiliation and incoherence. Time without lies. Communication without words where eyes and determination speak in place of spoken words. Yet the presence of childhood hides in a corner. It is time to say good-bye. Babble and tears are the lan-

guage of my dreams, and the song of my heartbeat.

The sun in Mexico was heavenly that winter and I spent hours outside on the balcony and ended up with a deep, glorious tan.

Returning to the States from Mexico, I went through Louisiana and at one stop the border patrol came aboard. I was pulled off the bus as an illegal. My suntan and shaggy hair got me in trouble. I got a bit insulted and "uppity" when I was pushed against the side of the bus.

"Listen to my voice," I said. "Can you hear Iowa? There is no Mexico there. I am an American citizen."

Border patrol roughly asked for my passport.

"I don't need a passport," I said. "I am an American citizen."

Fortunately, I had a passport, obtained when I went to Europe with my parents. I was let go, but I never forgot the incident; it made me realize the Gestapo mentality was not limited to Germany, and no matter who you were, you were vulnerable and at the mercy of the authorities, especially if you were young.

Shopped yesterday for wine at the friendly

little store in Alexandria. Wondered where Ann was. Couldn't remember my usual selections, so I asked the young man there if he remembered my favorites. He did and we picked four bottles.

Checking out, the clerk wanted my address to add to the new computer. I stumbled, restarted, but couldn't remember for sure what it was. Finally I recalled my driver's license had the address. This was the first time my memory tumbled in public on such a common piece of information. I was embarrassed at the stumble. One thing I have done to lessen problems has been to inform the people with whom I do business that I have Alzheimer's.

I hear the bird sing its staccato song outside my bedroom window, a dark morning with mind jumbled in a junkyard piled with anxiety and broken thoughts from a runaway mind.

My spelling has become so bad it is difficult to decipher the meaning in my sentences. Even small, familiar words such as "blew" are beyond my recall and have to be painfully sought in the dictionary. It is torture to go though this, and slow. I am fifty-eight years old, but my mind is determined to

make me regress to a child of few words —
and worse.

During my wandering days after high
school, I became interested in writing plays
and thought a little acting might be interesting and useful. I spent a brief few
summer-stock weeks in the unpaid boon-
docks, residing in a hot and airless hotel
room in the small town of Frederick, Maryland.

A different play was presented each week
with rehearsals each day and shows at
night. I, the kid who avoided public
speaking in high school because I was too
afraid to stand up and talk, knew I was
never going to be an actor.

An early wastrel summer was ahead, but
I stayed long enough in Frederick summer
stock to miss the annual trek to Eldora. A
summer in the tall corn of Iowa was no romance anymore. By skipping the Iowa vacation, I also missed visits to the dentist,
another annual event during the family's
two weeks in Eldora.

Almost from the first day, I was unhappy
with my choice of summer-stock play. I
had small bit parts and roustabout chores.
I couldn't remember lines or I got them
confused and the actors tried to circle

around and get me back to the two pages I left out. I was an unhappy, tortured fool in bit parts, strutting before a nearly empty house when I wanted to be a writer not an actor.

After I was certain my parents and sister were on their way to Iowa, I slipped off in the dark, leaving behind the actors from New York and the eager young local women with tight bosoms who ached for a chance in the limelight. For me, at that time, the summer trips to Iowa were pilgrimages to a past of manicured memories and a circumscribed life unchanged from the days before my parents were born.

With my failing memory every day begins new — and often ends that way, unable to negotiate a past as short as twelve hours.

Strange things are happening. I blew up suddenly this morning with surprising force and frustration. The cause? The newspaper had not arrived. It brought loud anger and tears in a smoky explosion of uncontrolled emotion.

Little things wear down my emotional equilibrium. First vocabulary fractures; then my emotions explode like snowflakes in an angry blizzard.

I live a new life of slow motion, stumbling with lost confidence. New things are torturous, confusing, and hard to understand. Even the old stuff of my life is not always familiar but with time and patience it is often recognizable. My eyes tear for no reason and I explode, when in better times I might have laughed. Send me away. I cannot stand to live in this dying body with its floating alphabet. I do not want to see the life of my future.

As I lay awake this morning in 4 a.m. darkness, a light show began its yellow glow on the wall opposite me. Large splotches of yellow flitted before me, flickering from wall to ceiling. I thought the source might be car lights outside but there were no automobiles on the street. The yellow patches acted as if they were controlled from outside my mind but it was probably all in my head. There was no source of light in the room and every time I blinked the yellow splotch jerked to a new nervous home on the wall.

I lay alone and insignificant, aware and unaware, as yellow discs danced around the room. They snapped off and on in large, torn shapes, each one unique. The torn yellow reflections continued for several minutes and disappeared as I became more interested in their presence. It was a frightening way to awaken and I slept no more.

Was I given a glimpse of the biological war inside my brain? Did I witness a barrage of tiny cells die inside my brain in the yellow flare of battle? Were these peculiar apparitions warnings of tomorrow? What generated this magical reflection of the fires burning in the holocaust of my brain? New mysteries. No real apparitions yet.

. . . .

Joyce and I met over the counter in the art department of a large dry goods store in the early 1960s. Day after day I showed up and hung around to tell her fanciful and bizarre stories. I lived at home under worrying pressure from my parents wanting to know what their only son was going to do with himself. I was engaged in reading books of little socially redeeming value, making pottery, and trying to find my legs in the world of writing.

Joyce also lived at home and attended the Corcoran School of Art in Washington, DC. She was way ahead of me in art and in life. She already had a little car; I still rode a bike.

Before long she was picking me up on

her way home after work as I walked along Wilson Boulevard. We talked, and ate drive-in hamburgers almost every night and went out on dates.

Soon my parents soured of my wastrel ways and prodded me to get a job. I found one in a military uniform shop and quickly rented a place of my own, a one-bedroom apartment in Buckingham, one of the first apartment complexes in Arlington. Presents were in order on moving day, and Joyce gave me a lusty unclothed female mannikin from the throwaway pile in the basement of the department store where she worked. I placed it in the entryway to the apartment as naked as it was on arrival.

It was a strange way to begin a relationship but before long we talked of marriage. When it looked as if I might be drafted into the ugly Vietnam War (I was classified 1AO, a conscientious objector), we decided to marry. Married men were exempt from the draft then.

I met Joyce's parents for the first time when we told them of our decision to marry. I was given a stunning welcome by Joyce's mother, who took a cue from my last name and called me a "dirty wop."

We married anyway and Joyce moved

into my little apartment. At night we slept on a narrow day bed in the living room. Above us her caged bird watched the goings-on. The bedroom was filled with clay dust and pottery equipment; it was where I kept my homemade potter's kick wheel. By then Joyce had a wonderful job as an airline reservationist, a position that made possible a whirlwind vacation to England and Scotland. Before long our son-to-be, Francesco, caught us by surprise.

I am forced into old age against my will and I am full of rage.

When I travel to familiar places, I have always been able to visualize a crude map with all the turns for that specific journey courtesy of my brain. This attribute of memory provided reassurance of my ability to arrive at my destination without trouble. My brain is becoming shy with sharing this information with me.

A recent fishing trip with Francesco brought this new deficit to me powerfully. We had to wing the four-hour round-trip without maps. I had driven to Mossy Creek many times over the years, but I could no longer trace the way with my mental map before the trip. Francesco had been there several times but after we started he confessed he didn't remember the way. I had not forgotten completely, it was just difficult to locate the place in my brain where the information was stored. It was an interesting experiment in navigation.

I don't know how long I will be able to retrieve stored memory like this. For now I have found a risky way around the trash pile of dead cells in my brain. Yet, I cannot stop wondering when my internal roads will have too many detour signs to make it possible for me to depend on them to take me to where I want to go.

I live on the edge of fear and insecurity and I am filled with uncertainty.

Alzheimer's has made me wary and cunning. I cannot hide from the sun. Now I expose myself for all to see in nakedness and uncertain pain. You are only a blur though my tear-soaked eyes.

───────

One of the most exciting developments in neuroscience research during the past 10 years has been the refinement of techniques that allow scientists to visualize the activity and interactions of particular brain regions as they are used during cognitive operations such as memorizing, recalling, speaking, reading, learning, and other sorts of information processing. This window on the living brain can help scientists measure early changes in brain function or structure to identify those individuals who are at risk of Alzheimer's disease even before they develop the symptoms of the disease. These imaging techniques include photon emission tomography (PET) scans and single photon emission computed tomography (SPECT), which produce "maps" of the brain that give information about activity in particular regions as a person responds to a task or stimuli, and magnetic resonance imaging (MRI), which provided a way to look at the size and characteristics of brain structures.

— "PROGRESS REPORT ON
ALZHEIMER'S DISEASE,"
NATIONAL INSTITUTE ON AGING, 1999

———

Often when I awaken in the dusty morning light, the new day I see around me is patterned in tiny square checks through which I see the world. I blink my eyes but the images before me remain. It is as if I am looking close-up through an old screen door. The precision of the tiny checks makes me think I am awakening in some kind of cell, a prisoner behind minute, rigid crisscross bars. Before long the apparition disappears and the world becomes clear and normal as the sun comes up. Is this another signal from the war in my brain where I am on the losing side in a battle with Alzheimer's?

Mornings begin with tears and unfamiliar sightings. I am losing familiarity with myself.

Researchers at the Mayo Clinic have conducted several important studies in the use of MRI to measure shrinkage in the volume of the hippocampus. The initial studies were cross-sectional studies, which compared groups of individuals with various levels of mental function, from healthy to diagnosed Alzheimer's. In their newest study, the team actually followed a group of men and women with mild cognitive impairment over time to test the hypothesis that MRI-based measurements of hippocampal volume could predict the risk of future development of Alzheimer's. The team followed the patients for nearly 3 years, providing annual exams and tests of mental function. Twenty-seven of the 80 patients with mild cognitive impairment developed dementia over the course of the study, and the investigators found that there was indeed a clear association between hippocampal shrinkage at the beginning of the study in these patients and later conversion to Alzheimer's.

— "PROGRESS REPORT ON
ALZHEIMER'S DISEASE,"
NATIONAL INSTITUTE ON AGING, 1999

The sun is shining and warm spring air swirls around me as I sit on a large, rough stone. It is a beautiful, life-affirming day and I am a breath away from tears.

These were warm, wonderful times for Joyce and me in the apartment on George Mason Drive. Joyce was an airline reservationist and I worked in a picture frame shop and made pottery in the bedroom.

Pottery was something I began in the family house on 9th Street. I had great expectations of making a career out of mud, one of life's first and most endearing materials. I began by digging heavy yellow clay from the open bank along Four-Mile Run, the little creek I could see from my bedroom window on 9th Street. I dried it, pounded it into smooth dust, added other materials, and tried to throw pots, as the instruction books called the process of making pottery.

After the move to the apartment, my handmade wheel, on which the first pots were made, gave way to a more efficient electric model with a sturdy metal frame. It was this wheel, along with more sophisticated "dirt," that found itself in the basement of our house on 26th Street. It was during this time I discovered Edna Lee and her pottery gallery on the border of Alexandria and Arlington that everybody called Arlandria.

For a while, my unemployed self had a Saturday job in the basement of Lee's gallery. My job was to mix different dry clay and wet it. This was heavy, dirty work and the mixing was the most arduous. After the clay was mixed it sat for a week to allow the excess water to rise; then the clay was wedged by hand, pushing the air out of it to make it workable and smooth. The basement had lights but the work was tiring and I was always glad to come out of the earth and into the sunlight.

It was at Edna Lee's gallery that I met Dick Lafeen, a potter, artist, and teacher. I made some money posing as a Christ figure in a painting Lafeen painted one summer. All the artists I met wanted to help me, and Lafeen showed me many techniques in making pottery. I remember watching the potter create a huge flawless, thin-walled bowl. As the clay spun on the wheel, it rose like magic in Lafeen's hands, a living thing springing from a whirling disk, a colossus, beautiful and round with the subtle marks of the maker's finger-prints on it forever. Later, I saw the piece in Lee's gallery and it was decorated with a subtle, multicolored glaze that shimmered in the light and took my breath away.

On a pleasant, sunny day like this several years from now, I will die with no sense of what is happening and surrounded by mourners who can know nothing of my inner travail, a pain I will never be able to utter in my Alzheimer's silence.

I learned much about modern medical technology in the last year. I like best the part where you lie down in a semidark room and snooze inside an MRI or PET machine, massive devices emitting strange noises, although it is a very expensive nap. I like less the medical stuff where you take your clothes off and some guy tickles you where you thought it was private. There is a lot less of that with Alzheimer's because the interest is at the other end of the body where the brain lives, and that is fine with me.

In mid-February, eleven months after I begin this Alzheimer's audacity, I underwent another drowsy test, my first PET brain scan. PET stands for positron emission tomography, a high-tech machine to look inside a brain. It makes snapshots of what is in there. Eventually I received two beautiful sheets of negatives with little pictures of my brain.

Within a few weeks of the scan, Dr. Blanchfield explained it to me. She told it simply with a kindness that was straightforward and sympathetic. The dark stuff on the little pictures of my brain was good; the white or light-colored stuff was not, because it signaled something had been there and was gone. It was the opposite of what I had thought when I first saw the pictures.

John D. Rauth, Jr., who actually interpreted the complex imaging, explained it this way in a letter to Dr. Blanchfield:

"The patient is a fifty-eight-year-old male with memory and speech problems. His dementia is clinically more progressive than expected. An MRI performed on 3/11/99 was normal."

The PET scan revealed, according to Dr. Rauth, that "there is decreased activity involving the left parietal region bilaterally, left side more so than the right side. Also, there is decreased activity involving the temporal lobes, again left side more so than the right side. These findings are most consistent with early Alzheimer's disease."

This came as little surprise to me. My antenna had already picked this up. As I wrote this little book I encountered increased difficulty with language and loss of vocabulary, increased misspellings, and difficulty in organizing thoughts and sentences. I concluded my brain was under siege from Alzheimer's at a quick march. In some crazy way it is good to have my own assumptions reinforced, although this was one of the few times I wish my intuition was wrong.

Memory is seduction.

There was a little newspaper called *under-*

ground back in the sixties and it was all mine. It was written and put together in the house on 26th Street, a domicile often filled with laughter, politics, music, and strange people. A few newsstands in Washington, New York, and San Francisco sold the paper. Joyce, baby Francesco, and I hawked the paper on street corners and college campuses in Washington.

These were the beginning days of U.S. involvement in Vietnam, as politics began to overcome culture and music, and paranoia became the food of conquest.

Carl Bernstein, then a reporter for the *Washington Post* before his exposé of Watergate with Bob Woodward, made *underground*, my newspaper, locally famous with an article. The *Post*'s attention was focused on an incident at American University in which a school official tried to keep Joyce from selling papers with little Francesco in her arms. The incident quickly grew as students surrounded them with free press rhetoric.

Publicity about the event brought a series of hate calls and threats. It also increased the number of friends and strangers who came by to serenade us with tunes on spoons and nose flutes or to "yak" about books or the state of the nation, or to find out whether we were wife swappers. Joyce and I loved company so much and had so little money that almost anyone who knocked on the door was admitted, even a disheveled man with an alcoholic pallor who kept dropping his pants.

One of the first strangers to whom we opened our door was a large man who came to sell cemetery plots. The usual misunderstanding between salesman and potential customer occurred. He thought we wanted to buy; we thought he was entertainment. All I remember of him are his fingers. On one hand fingers were tattooed with the word "LOVE" and on the other "HATE." It was an emblematic marriage of words for the times.

Little Francesco crawled through it all. What else could he do? There was no television in the house.

Since December 1999, every three months or so Noah Adams of National Public Radio arrives at our farm in Loudoun County, Virginia, with two colleagues, producer Lisa Harmon and soundman Drew Reynolds. We sit down in Francesco and Tammy's living room for an interview about how Joyce, Francesco, and I are getting along with Alzheimer's. Noah asks questions in the manner of a kindly doctor. Here are some of the letters that arrived at the Washington, DC, headquarters of NPR after the second interview:

I am writing to thank you for your story about the DeBaggio family of Virginia and their struggle with early Alzheimer's disease. As a clinical neuro-psychologist, I am very familiar with the symptoms of Alzheimer's disease and its debilitating effect on everyday functioning. Your story, however, reminded me of how Alzheimer's disease feels to those who cope with it on a daily basis. I was touched by the honesty of Mr. DeBaggio and his family, and I commend them for allowing us all to share in their journey.

I am the son of a Parkinson's sufferer, a similarly debilitating neurological disease. I was struck by the many similarities between Mr. DeBaggio's mind-set and that of my father. Reflecting on Mr. DeBaggio's description of the transition from early "puzzlement" with his condition, to frustration and infuriation at the pace of its advance has really helped me better understand my father's situation as his condition worsens.

My dad was diagnosed with Alzheimer's 11 years ago in his early 50's. As horrible as the disease sounded when we first researched it, the reality has been even more cruel. After a few years, my dad was reduced from a loving, sharp-minded, and athletic man to an agitated, utterly helpless, distorted shell. My mom has been simply heroic in her care and advocacy for him and he gets the best care available. Yet it is hard to believe that he is not miserable. But, somehow, his humanity and goodness are still evident — in a sigh, a touch, or a look in the eye. And that is the hardest part of all.

In my opinion you have performed a disservice today in your follow-up interview with the DeBaggio family and early Alzheimer's disease. In your earlier interview, I believe that some documentation that Mr. DeBaggio had the disease was provided. Little background was provided today, and the interview appeared to be an attempt to present manifestations of the progression of the disease. What is frightening is the apparent normal behavior of this man.

In its earliest form, manifestations of Alzheimer's disease may be subtle. Emotional behavior, forgetting names, confusion, and frustration in operating telephones may reflect early Alzheimer's or overlap normal behavior or normal aging. The fact that Mr. DeBaggio believes he suffers from the disease may increase his anxiety and exaggerate his symptoms, as it will normal individuals. I wonder how much anxiety you have created and how many people will wonder whether they have early Alzheimer's disease after listening to this interview?

Are we born with a fear of our bodies? Could that be why we pay so little attention to what is inside and so many hours are spent pampering the exterior and festooning it with colorful threads? We breathe without awareness. Not until something goes cockeyed wrong inside do we become aware there is an inside to look after, an interior for the mind, as well as the arteries. There is so much to know, so little time, and we pay so little attention to an elbow.

Maybe it is good we are so body ignorant. If we spent time trying to understand what goes on inside, we'd get nothing done. Might not be a bad idea, doing less and shaping our lives on nothingness.

One day there was a knock on the door of the house on 26th Street. I opened it to find a wiry, aging man before me. He came from New York where he read a copy of *underground*. He stepped inside. Thus did Joyce and I begin a fast, unbelievable ride on the politics of the absurd.

Austin said he was an advertising executive from New York, preparing his run for vice-presidency of the United States. Of course he wanted help, bodies if not money.

That first day Joyce and I listened and laughed as Austin recounted wacky stories from his campaign. After a few hours of nonstop talk, it was clear he was a modern Don Quixote without a biographer. When we got weary, we bunked him with baby Francesco, although Austin was provided a bed of his own.

A few weeks later he appeared again. He stood before the open door holding a woman's leather Indian costume for Joyce. He had a male costume full of feathers for himself. Joyce became Princess Summer-

Fall-Winter-Spring; Austin was Chief Burning Wood.

His idea was to do a little politicking and hell-raising on Capitol Hill. In preparation for his political appearance on the Hill, he sent a series of outlandish letters to favored salons.

The historic morning was cold but there is warmth in humor, especially when there are enough bellies laughing. Baby Francesco was along, probably the youngest political hanger-on in history. The first stop was uneventful, except Austin was unable to talk with his congressman. We walked around the corner to another office. This time we were greeted at the door, but the entrance was blocked by a large man, a congressional aide.

As the day wore on, a contingent of Capitol Hill police attached itself to our foursome. The men in blue never joined the "Indians" in the elevators. One time Austin waited a few seconds after the elevator doors closed and then pushed the "open" button. Before us we saw the Capitol Hill policemen running in all directions, sliding on the slick marble floors, trying to regain traction to carry them up stairways and down, in an effort to reach the next floor when the elevator stopped.

None of the congressmen met with Chief Burning Wood and Princess Summer-Fall-Winter-Spring with her little papoose or the lanky, black-bearded guy taking notes.

Austin was overwhelmed by his day on Capitol Hill. On his way around the Capitol Beltway in the dark, he missed the turn to New York several times. Afterward he said he continued to circle Washington to put a hex on Congress.

Some days it seems I live in two worlds. In one I am afflicted with Alzheimer's, gasping as words slip though my lips with effort and suffering imprecision. This is the world in which I have to tell my companion I can't remember the word to make the sentence.

In the other, slower world where I write on paper or directly on the computer, vocabulary is more fluid and I often surprise myself when the perfect word finds its way into the sentence without effort. This has puzzled me from the first sentence I wrote for this book. It is only now, eight months later, I begin to see more clearly how necessary it is to slow the pace to achieve a former normality.

The reason for the difference may be

that speaking is performance, a public act with nervous tension, while writing, although it may carry the same words and meaning, is private, slow paced, and more amenable to revision. The narrow edge between writing and speaking makes a larger difference in the world than I imagined before Alzheimer's. Perhaps it also has to do with seeing the written words. Spoken words are born and die quickly. When written, words are created more deliberately, and may call upon a larger part of the brain.

My days are gone, forgotten in a garbage bag of the soul. Only empty flesh remains where there was once a man with a mind filled with dreams.

The day after I was diagnosed with Alzheimer's, my first thought when I awoke was of suicide. It appeared to be a logical thing to contemplate. I was facing a difficult, slow decline, leading to eventual loss of nearly everything human beings value, ending finally as a near-vegetable rotting in the sun. Most important, my early demise saves thousands of dollars spent on my care as I deteriorate. I didn't want Joyce to end a pauper or have Francesco lose the farm.

I talked to Joyce about my thoughts carefully. It is to her I defer because she carries the burden of my care. I saw tears tease her eyes but her voice was clear and emphatic. She was against the plan. She wanted me around as long as possible in any condition but dead.

I deferred to her wishes. It is for her I live now; there is nothing else for me. A real life has expectations and dreams, and mine are gone, unless you include my desire to catch another large trout on Mossy Creek. I no longer easily remember what day it is and I have trouble remembering routines I have followed for decades. The savageness of my out-of-control body is a surprise to me and its quick ugliness frightens me. Some part of me will live through it until the last day, but the young Tommy I was forty-five years ago is quickly dying and is more a memory for others now.

As I write this, tears suddenly begin to flow from my eyes and I choke in spasms of grief. The past surprises me with emotion I never realized was there. The tears remind me of how little time I have left with these memories.

More and more I am unconsciously mixing words that have similar sounds: our and out, would and wood, me and be, to name a few. This leaking alphabet of reality is something I might have expected in speech, not in writing.

I look to the future and see myself in a state of not dying but without life, an unseen cripple. I am a place barren of memory. I can see myself in a mirror but I do not recognize the image in the glass. The world around me is filled with secrets, entombed in lost memory. I stand on the corner, waiting for the light to change. Without memory I am unknown to myself, lost in an anxiety of darkness.

I found myself strangely silent at Joyce's Sunday birthday party. The search for words was too great a struggle. Silence hid my handicap and made life easier. Alzheimer's is making me mute out of necessity. I will save my spoken words to decorate these pages.

Life has slowed as I watch Alzheimer's take over. Even the simplest tasks become laborious with a hesitating rhythm. No longer does my mind run me. I must wait for it to catch up before I know where I am.

. . . .

How did I find my way to a flophouse in the county seat town of Peru, Indiana? It was an act of desperation; I was out of money, broke by my desire to publish truth. I was anxious for a job in journalism and I pored over job ads in trade papers. The *Peru Daily Tribune* was one of the many newspapers to which I sent a résumé. After an interview, I got the job.

Before I settled down in Indiana, a trip to Iowa to see my parents was in order. They moved back to Eldora a few weeks after Francesco's birth and they prayed for a visitation of the little one. On the way back from our visit, Joyce dropped me in Peru where I rented a dark, smelly flophouse room opposite the newspaper, and looked for accommodations for my family. Joyce and Francesco went back to Arlington to pack.

Soon I found a place to live in the upper floor of a generous duplex and started painting the dingy walls. The biggest drawback of the apartment was a staircase connecting the upstairs and downstairs kitchens. Later it was common to see the landlord's shirttail disappearing down the steps when Joyce and I came home.

For mental succor I befriended the town librarian, Dave Bucove, an Easterner who knew the town and its foibles. Dave was instrumental in having all my *underground* papers microfilmed.

I discovered Paul Kelly, a curmudgeon with an acid sense of humor, at a town festival. A displaced Chicagoan, he was the last vestige of the circus in Peru. The barn on his farm swayed with the weight of elephants and their babies. He was outspoken, to put it mildly. Although the town claimed the birthplace of Cole Porter, Kelly's description was not lyrical. He dubbed Peru the last cemetery in the United States with lights and running water. Francesco fell in love with Kelly's ponies one afternoon. Joyce primed her house plants with Kelly's zoo-do.

A tip came my way from the local head of the NAACP. A restaurant in town was notorious for barring blacks, I was told. An attempt to eat there was going to be made by the local members of the NAACP. It was time Joyce and I ate out and we went to dinner at the restaurant in question. A short time after we sat down, two black couples I recognized walked in and were seated near me. There was great relief when they started to eat. It was the first time I was happy not to write a story.

One day a reporter came in and told me some scuttlebutt at the barber shop was spreading a rumor I was a communist. The postman tipped them; I received a suspicious, large package in the mail every day. I laughed. The large packages were the *Congressional Record*, the official document of the U.S. Congress.

For all my faults, I began to enjoy my work, but it was not long before the routine chafed my creativity. I tired of making the rounds to the police department, the sheriff's office, and the fire department. But quirky stories always turned up to explain the town in new ways. I loved these tales for their humanity and they hung in my memory. One morning the police blotter noted a theft at a gas station. The money was left, but the toilet was stolen. Another day, firemen wondered how a man and a woman, in broad daylight, used the telephone booth in front of the firehouse for a toilet.

It is hard to be embarrassed when you can't remember who you are, what you said, or where you are going.

Almost every minute of the day is distorted by the struggle to reclaim lost words and the frustrating search to communicate. It is a battle with little purpose. No matter how hard I try, this is one battle I will not win without a miracle.

There are days when I become lost in the destructive power of Alzheimer's.

As I lay awake this morning in 4 a.m. darkness, I was treated to a light show. A series of yellow images with edges torn in irregular patterns began to flash slowly before me as I stared at the wall opposite me. They danced before my eyes as if they were projected on the wall but there was no source of light for them. They could only be generated in my mind but they were as real as if Picasso was squirting the wall with random objects painted in yellow. I lay there alone and insignificant and for several minutes the yellow-lit objects snapped on and off in different places on the wall.

My first thought was that these images were reflections of the fires burning in the holocaust of my brain. It was no mysterious apparition, according to my doctor.

It was just another manifestation of Alzheimer's, a warning light on the way to loneliness and hell.

———

The time must come to all of us, who live long, when memory is more important than prospect.
— VISCOUNT GREY
OF FALLODON, 1930, IN *FLY FISHING*

———

Familiar habits peel away and are lost from memory. Everything is becoming new with an aspect of unfamiliarity. There is the confusion of the object seen for the first time. I am in an unfamiliar world but I stand still.

I rattle my cage but no one comes to feed me.

For the last fifteen years, I have walked the same three miles every morning. When I began, the landscape was familiar. In the last few years, major changes have taken place and now the feeling of a small town is gone and in its place are twenty-story highrise buildings for living and work. My little world is becoming crowded as these new structures shoulder their way down the streets toward me. I walk through the streets now remembering when I was a boy building model railroads and playing ball in the middle of 9th Street. I wonder where the sun has gone and what has happened to the world I knew.

As I walked yesterday in fresh, early morning, a woman pushing a stroller with a little girl in it passed me on the right. I am a fast walker and I am usually the one passing people. I watched the woman pushing the stroller pull away from me, bending her body forward to lower her profile. I stopped for a moment to look at the progress of a new office building and when I turned back to the sidewalk, the woman pushing the stroller was gone. I looked around when I got to the place she had been but there was nothing there but her hurried memory. Had she ever been there? I was uncertain whether I really saw her.

A call came to the *Peru Daily Tribune* from the *Wilmington News-Journal* in Delaware. The company was searching for journalists with experience on small papers who were ready to move to larger organizations. I was surprised my editor in Peru told me of the opportunity, but I quickly understood it was a subtle invitation to move.

I knew nothing of the searing riots and

mass arrests in Wilmington after Dr. Martin Luther King's assassination, nor did I know about the city's struggle under martial law and curfews for nine months.

I planned to fly on the *News-Journal*'s ticket, but missed the plane and drove through the night to Delaware. I arrived in time for the interview. Upon returning to Indiana, I got a call telling me I had the job. The packing began immediately.

Soon I was sitting at a desk in the *News-Journal*'s scruffy newsroom. I was filled with first-day jitters and tingling excitement. My first job was writing obituaries of local soldiers killed in the Vietnam War. The routine work bored me. Making phone calls to the families of the dead soldiers was emotionally difficult but I worked up a spiel to make it easier, something about writing a tribute to a fallen son or husband.

Soon I realized I had just traded a job with a set routine and familiar faces for work that was empty one minute and boring the next. What I liked least was the lack of control over my choice of work. I learned to accept as punishment interviews with strange people standing in vest-pocket parks at 2 a.m.

The stories I most enjoyed reporting

were those I sought myself. These were in poor parts of town where there was hunger, anger, and discrimination. It wasn't long before I hunted my own stories and worked on them at home. I polished one on the University of Delaware's involvement in the Vietnam War. When I saw it later, it had been edited with notations in different colored inks. The DuPont family owned the newspaper through a holding company and board members were given opportunities to shape stories to protect their interests; the color of ink secretly identified each commentator.

When I left after 180 frustrating days on the job, the newspaper's editor, Dixie Sanger, had me in for a quiet talk. He asked me not to "slam the door too hard" when I left. Of course I didn't listen to talk like that. After walking out of his office I immediately wrote an article for an antipoverty organization about my experience. I called it "180 Days in a House of Ill Repute." Subtlety has never been my forte.

Almost every minute of the day is destroyed by the struggle to reclaim lost words in my search to communicate. It is a losing battle, but I will sing until no word is left. Alzheimer's is making me mute.

I sometimes stumble through my shrinking vocabulary, lost in a world of detached alphabet, unsure and waiting for the next smirk of evil. I know where this leads, even through the blurred vision of tears.

When you shut your eyes, the world goes black. That was the way it was for me until recently. Now it is black when I shut my eyes during the day, but at night there is a change. Instead of black, a panoply of colors, with a subtle sparkle, rolls before my eyes. Gradually the speed of the roll slows and I am quickly asleep in minutes. This is one of the pleasant aspects of sharing a bed with Alzheimer's.

What am I doing here?

I launched yet another ill-starred newspaper, a monthly called the *Wilmington Independent.* For an office, I used a spare room in the apartment; what little money Joyce and I saved funded it. Little equipment was needed: a typewriter, some glue, and knowledge of newspaper layout. There were many newspapers printing tabloids for others then, and now.

One of the first stories I came across was the treatment of inmates in Delaware prisons. I had many sources inside and outside prison and word got back to me of mistreatment. One of the most notorious punishments was tying nearly naked prisoners to steel beds and leaving them there for hours.

I lacked entrée but I learned the Delaware Human Relations Commission planned a visit to the prison. I hitched a ride with the head of the Commission, who was worried about prison conditions. The two-person Commission had free run of the facility and talked to many inmates.

Delaware had a long history of mistreatment of prisoners and there was great debate, as late as the 1960s, about bringing back the whipping post. Delaware was the last state to use this medieval torture and there was still serious debate about reinstating the punishment.

The story I wrote for my newspaper did not please the penal community, at least those not behind the bars. As I discovered later, it was responsible for keeping me out of prison. Two years later, while working as an editor for the *Delaware Spectator*, a weekly published by an antipoverty group,

I attempted to interview prisoners in the correctional center in Syrma, Delaware. It was then I learned I had been barred from entry to any Delaware prison because of the earlier article.

Sometimes a telephone call could ignite a story for the *Independent*. This one was from a salesperson cold-calling potential buyers of oceanfront property for Ocean Pines, a Boise Cascade Company. I asked an innocent question: did the company permit blacks? "No," the caller said.

I jumped at the story. I knew such exclusion was illegal. Of course, I wanted a rep to visit me. When she arrived the next evening, I pressed her about the company's failure to maintain equal housing when its brochure said it was a "fair housing community." She said it was a lie. Loss of employment was the penalty for salespeople who invited black couples to purchase property. If any salesperson let them through, a method was concocted to bar their entry through a system of disqualifying checks.

Within a few weeks of publication of the story, a Washington lawyer called me. He told me he represented a black Delaware couple going before a hearing judge in

Washington, DC. They had been selected out by Boise Cascade. The lawyer wanted me to testify. I went to Washington, waited outside the hearing room, but when my time to testify came, lunch was called. The hearing never resumed; Boise Cascade, with powerful influence in Washington, decided to settle, a clever way for powerful, well-connected firms to hide their misdeeds.

I managed to ruffle many feathers with the *Independent*, but lacked the money for the long haul necessary to maintain a muckraking newspaper in a company town like Wilmington.

I am amazed when I can remember something that happened an hour ago.

. . . .

My Alzheimer's is still subtle and not yet crippling. Yet I can feel the desire to drop my pants and masturbate in public and indulge in other behavior typical of diminished inhibition. And this is happening at the same time my sexual drive has begun to stall. Obviously, in many ways, I am regressing toward a childhood I never knew.

Alzheimer's is catching, often passed from parent to child through faulty genes.

320

***

Dreaming is something that disappeared from my nightlife some years ago, perhaps with the surreptitious start of Alzheimer's destruction. I have recently had presleep moments of rolling color before my eyes and hallucinations, but last night topped them all.

It began halfway through my night's sleep. I was gripped with fearsome emotion. I ran in the dark of my dream trying to hide, from what I did not know. I ran in fear from what, the fear that haunts us all in night sweat. I was lost. I knocked on doors and I tapped on windows. No one helped me. I was terrified.

I awoke suddenly, shaking from the nightmare. Joyce tried to calm me. She had heard me screaming in my sleep and came into the room to see what was happening.

I am lost. I am lost. It was a wretched litany. My breath came like that of a frightened child, afraid of the dark and wary of a world not understood.

With Joyce's arms around me for comfort, I began mumbling, "I am home. I am home." I needed assurance I was no longer in the terrible dream in a broken world out of order, licked by chaos. I continued to murmur rhythmically, "I'm home, I'm home," like a little child.

I have never had such a frightening experience, except, perhaps, that night when my parents slipped out, leaving the apartment door open, to sit and talk with their friends across the hall, and I awoke with fear and loneliness in my crib.

In my sleep, did my beleaguered memory cause me to relive the moment long ago when a two-year-old screamed until his parents returned to the sound of his abandonment?

Joyce and I made friends everywhere we went in Wilmington. We looked for people like ourselves, "peaceniks" and civil rights activists. Through them, and a circle of Quakers, I discovered on the city's edge the still, quiet woods overlooking a green meadow beside a little brook. It was here that a breakaway group of Quakers met every Sunday morning. Joyce and I knew little about Quaker services, but we were friends with several of the members of the group and we were invited to participate. It was here that we felt the calm life force inhabiting Ethel Snyder, a woman as close to sainthood as I had ever met.

The Sunday meetings in the meadow were built on Quaker practice with some outdoor refinements. Everybody sat in a circle on the grass and held hands, happy in their humanity and the rich silence inhabiting the group. After a while, in Quaker style, a member of the circle talked into the silence. Soon another voice spoke. They expressed deep-earth thoughts, not prayers.

Afterward the kids played and there was fine socializing. It was something Joyce and I never experienced again and it left a mark on us that we still carry.

I had a wonderful lunch on the Alzheimer's Association, local chapter, today. They have a plan to make me into a poster boy and I am willing to let them use me. Anything to bring attention and money to help end this scourge is all right with me. I squirm at having a spotlight shine on me, but it is just a means to something greater, helping other people whose lives are also twisted in the torturous claws of Alzheimer's.

After I got home from the lunch, I had an idea and called the local chapter. As the receptionist answered, my mind went blank and I couldn't remember why I called or the name of the person I wanted to talk to. I sputtered and the receptionist giggled hysterically, thinking, perhaps, I was playing a joke.

I was breathlessly angry with myself. I have made it standard procedure lately to outline on paper what I want to say before I make a call so this does not happen. I became overconfident and made a fool of myself. By the time I hung up, I remembered why I called and dialed back without incident.

As new drugs to treat and even prevent Alzheimer's disease make their way through the pipeline, a basic medical issue has remained unresolved: how can doctors know which patient to medicate if they are not yet showing clear-cut symptoms?

Now researchers believe they may find an answer in the magnetic resonance imaging machines. The findings are reported in a new study paid for by the National Institute on Aging; it appears in the *Annals of Neurology.*

The scientists found some regions of the brain change size in patients in the early stages of Alzheimer's. When this happens, the warning signs are visible on an MRI. This may one day allow doctors to identify patients in early stages of Alzheimer's who could benefit from drugs as they become available. But, the lead researcher, Dr.

Marilyn S. Albert of Massachusetts General Hospital, cautioned that the technique needed much refinement.

"It's not there yet," she said, "and I don't want to mislead people."

The researchers — who are also from Brigham and Women's Hospital and from Harvard, Brandeis, and Boston Universities — were able to confirm earlier studies that found significant neuron loss in some parts of the brain during early Alzheimer's.

Over three years, the researchers studied 119 people with an average age in the early 70s, some healthy and others with mild memory problems. As subjects developed the disease, the researchers went back and reviewed their earlier MRIs.

In every case, they reported the MRI distinguished between healthy participants and those with mild Alzheimer's. Scans of the entorhinal cortex could detect a difference between healthy people and memory-impaired patients who went on to develop the disease.

One time in the good old days, my lawyer father told me he had been selected, along with many other men and women working in the government, to hide in secret concrete bunkers deep in Virginia's Blue Ridge Mountains and run the country during a potential war with the Soviet Union. I never understood why a lawyer working for the Bureau of Narcotics was needed in an underground bunker but it must have had something to do with the high potency medicines that might be needed and were regulated by his office.

The thought of his leaving me, my sister, and my mother, perhaps never seeing us again, must have made him shake with fear and sorrow. At my age, living underground sounded like fun. Newspapers of the times were full of stories of families so fearful of the possibility of conflagration they built underground bunkers in their backyards and stocked them with canned foods, matches, and spirit lamps. Air raid siren tests made the possibility seem even more real. The fear generated was palpable, but my father never took up residency underground and the rest of the fear that was generated soon evaporated and was forgotten.

The childhood wounds healed, and my dreams were less haunted by fear. Imagination soon replaced anxiety and I learned early its lonely, lovely powers.

Instead of focusing on the explosive reality of their time, my parents created for me and my sister a happier personal interval of their own imagining. This created optimism in us and a gentle narrative of childhood tranquility. They showed me the beauty of the cornfields of Iowa and the serenity of a small town called Eldora.

Soon enough I was scarred and uplifted, as were they, by the time of my time, a world of conflagration, disorder, hope, ugliness, great beauty, and unnecessary death. The imaginative world of kindness and promise they passed to me remained untouched by the ugliness of congested cities, immoral wars, and encompassing greed.

In the past, I was a man who did not move in his sleep. Lately I toss and turn on a disheveled bed. Night after night strange dreams inhabit my sleep, nights of lost wandering, terror, fear, and mysterious occurrences. These are dreams of confusion, deep, dreadful dreams I categorize as Alzheimer's experiences. In them the man I see is walking, wandering aimlessly, lost and fearful. I wake up screaming, fearing loss of control, hiccupping with fear, breathless with emotion. I feel myself dying night by night, as I mark off strange wads of wandering scattered in resistant sleep. My mind jumps as if a computer screen scrolled out of control. I am lost and afraid, headed for a hell imagined by a dyspeptic surrealist.

It's the lights again, always at night, the colored lights rolling in front of me too innocent to wonder. When I close my eyes, I am afraid the colors will roll before me. I am lost in nightmare, afraid to sleep, too tired to remember who I am. There is ugliness more but I am going to keep that secret by forgetting. Hide by the tree with me. Watch the little boy on the swing.

I can remember the skeleton but not the fleshy record that made it a man.

Memory has been abundant in the human family and even in other animals. I took it for granted until recently, as my recall began to sag and it became clear Alzheimer's was a dog nipping my toes. As disease subtly steals these sweet nuggets of the past, an unknown loneliness has taken hold. Where the past once bubbled with memories, it now has long breaks punctuated with nightmares instead of pleasant dreams. My past is disappearing, removed forever, a painful little pit of me lost forever. As I write, I must rely on notes taken a year ago as this project began. I am reminded now how sweet is memory, how comforting and important.

Memory is in the present, one minute at a time, and that is disappearing at an alarming rate. I am truly living in the present. My memory of yesterday is obliterated as I lived it; there is hardly a light to illuminate the long tunnel of yesterday. Most of my memory is obliterated the instant it is created.

Loneliness becomes physical, an ocean without foam or movement, a stagnant puddle. This loneliness creates a silence you can hear. The only way I have to preserve my memory now is to write. This book becomes my memory, the only record I have of these empty, dead days.

Life in me gradually seeps away as Alzheimer's gains control of my mind and body, chipping where I cannot watch. I am not yet a vegetable waiting to rot but I can feel the aura of death in the white hairs of my head and in every pore of my body.

There is a time in every life when this moment occurs — sometimes slowly, at other occasions almost instantly — and it creates an unsteady moment of revelation. This is the first time I have truly faced the idea of death. Previously I have had fleeting knowledge. I have watched parents and grandparents age and stumble into unrewarded dotage. The most intimate I have been with death was watching Joyce's mother slowly deteriorate into nothingness, slimming to the bone, each day becoming weaker. Even that did not prepare me. Even the waiting for her last breath as she lay helpless and silent on her bed in a darkened room. I heard no screaming words, no complaints or gurgles; the ordinary continued without my awareness of the internal doubt and trembling. It was not until several days after I forgot where I was headed while driving the car and became unreasonably emotional and agitated that death, my death, began to live in me.

. . . .

The woods above the meadow were fine cover and a place of secrets. The privacy of the tall, clustered trees created a secretive world. It was an ideal place to interview individuals frightened for their lives by knowledge they had.

One afternoon I took a walk in the woods with a woman I knew. We walked the rutted yellow clay path together as the dappled light slid through the leafy tree branches. She told me secrets about an underworld of threats and violence, peopled by men in places of security and honor, including the police department.

"Doris" began her double life the day she realized too many of her friends had fallen victims to the needle's euphoria. One night, an hour before a large heroin shipment was due, she phoned a police captain, her main contact. She told him about the drug shipment. "Keep in touch," he said. "I can't do anything now. I'll wait for you to call me with more information." Doris went to the delivery site and copied license numbers on cars outside the drug house. She telephoned her captain, but there was no answer. An official state car was involved in carrying the drugs, she said.

The more Doris saw, the more she came to believe a complex web held everything together. The whores, the pimps, the gamblers, the numbers writers, the rogue cops, the bootleggers, some politicians, government officials, and businessmen were all interconnected.

Before her story was published, she went into hiding in another state. I saw her once more. This time the underworld she worked was a spiritual one.

There are secrets in every town. Those

who know the secrets are few and they risk much, sometimes their lives, by sharing them with others.

Memory is a tricky, sometimes fickle, organ. Jane E. Brody of the *New York Times* in her "Personal Health" column of April 25, 2000, shed light on false memory enhancement, and its consequences.

"There is no question that the memory of traumatic events can sometimes become repressed," she wrote. "But there is also no question that many so-called recovered memories, particularly those involving allegations of childhood sexual abuse by a parent or other close relative, teacher or friend, are often fictions induced by the concerted efforts of a therapist who fosters a belief that becomes so deeply held it seems like a real memory."

"We don't know what percent of these recovered memories are real and what percent are pseudo-memories," said Dr. Harold Lief, a psychiatrist.

"A young woman in psychotherapy recovered the memory that at age 13 she was raped by her teacher, became pregnant and underwent an abortion," Brody wrote. "In fact, the woman had not reached puberty until 15, so the pregnancy was medically impossible."

"By asking a series of leading questions and by having a supposed 'witness' talk about the made-up experience," wrote Brody, "it is often possible to convince someone that the event actually happened. In one study, researchers easily convinced half the adult patients that they had been hospitalized in severe pain as children or that they had been lost in a shopping mall at age 5. Several people with these false memories provided detailed embellishments."

A study at Cornell University showed how easily children can be convinced fiction is reality. "Preschool children were asked weekly about whether a fictitious event had ever happened to them," Brody wrote. "By the 10th week, more than half reported it had happened and provided cogent details about it. In one experiment, interviewers told the children: 'Think real hard. Did you get your hand caught in a mousetrap and go to the hospital to get it off?' "

Dr. Stephen J. Ceci reported: "So compelling did the children's narrative appear that we suspect that some of the children had come to truly believe they had experienced the fictitious events. Neither parents nor researchers were able to convince 27 percent of the children that the events never happened."

Not long ago my mind was quick and sharp. Now it is a game of hide and seek. I feel something in my mind waiting on the edge of consciousness but it does not materialize; it hides from disclosure. My life is plump with moments of twisted awareness, moments when memory dies. Time has turned into a premonition instead of reality. Alzheimer's has given new meaning to the idea of having your head in the clouds.

Wilmington was more than Rodney Square and DuPont Castles in the leafy suburbs. There was the East Side, the place to escape, ringed by industry and filled with grief and struggle for life. Its lonely streets of fear were peopled with brazen, outspoken men like Tobe, Balagun, and Bill Young, saints if given a chance. But this was the place of original sin, a home where humans struggled to be good and survive with honor and were tricked into evil. Life here was short and unhappy, often ending with a bullet or an overdose. Those still luckily alive were often drafted into prison. This side of Wilmington was flooded with tears and anger.

The cancer holding the East Side hostage leaked everywhere and one day Joyce and I found it oozing into our house. Joyce went to an anti-war meeting at a friend's house. I was with little Francesco when the phone rang.

"Do you know where Joyce is?" the caller asked.

It was a strange way to start a conversation with a stranger. I had been wondering whether we were being watched; now I was certain. Was the telephone tapped as well?

"She's gone to a meeting," I said.

"Just about now she is naked and in bed with a buck-naked nigger football player," he said. I hung up the phone. I felt strange, as if I had just been violated. I was surprised someone watched the comings and goings at our apartment. When I told Joyce of the incident, she was upset that anyone thought she could be interested in a football player.

The police state began in the wake of riots after Dr. King was assassinated and wide latitude was granted the police and the military. After nine months of practice in martial law, the police state was no longer a shadow in America; it was reality.

Joyce and I went to a meeting of the White

People Coalition for Peace and Justice soon after we arrived in Delaware. It was here where we were enfolded in kindness, humanity, and sanity. We met Ruth, Vona, Harriet, and the earth-mother goddess of all, Ethel Snyder. It was here where a man was pointed out as an FBI informant. The FBI had a large presence in Wilmington and individuals were hired to bring them information.

Months later, I ran into that man at the grocery store. We chatted and the man asked me if I'd like to accompany him to a Ku Klux Klan rally in nearby Maryland. I immediately saw a story.

The Klan meeting was in a farmer's meadow. It was filled with white-sheeted, masked men and women. I stood back and watched as the man I knew as an FBI informant worked the crowds, getting whatever information interested J. Edgar Hoover. I may have ended up being the only name he could give up.

Years later I obtained my FBI file and my attendance at the Klan rally was duly noted. The name of the informant was blacked out on the paper, but not in my memory. It must have been difficult for the FBI to understand what a leftist journalist was doing at a Klan meeting. It was all grist for the police state. Whatever it cost to report on the whereabouts of Joyce and me, it was a waste of taxpayer money and a violation of our civil rights.

Although my memory is crumbling into obscurity, I am a memory for someone, living again in their recollection.

Once my days were bright with ideas and dreams, a butterfly of words dancing in the sun of certainty. Now a dull emptiness wraps its arms around me in a suffocating embrace. The words in my brain are silent, and the flood of sentences begins only when my pen unleashes a flood of writing memory. After so many years coddling words, it is now I realize writing carries the blood of memory.

As thoughts and ideas evaporate, sometimes more quickly than I can catch them, my enjoyment of life is shredded. This is a small part of what lies ahead.

When the brain loses its controls, memory sags and the simple becomes complex. I took it for granted; it never occurred to me how important the thing on top of my shoulders was. In the last year, I gained new respect for the brain and its twenty-four-hour work. It may be the hardest working thing on earth, the brain, and it comes free with designer colors on the package.

I never realized how important the brain was to the enjoyment of life. It is not just about remembering things; it is about where things are and how they work. It is about the retrieval of knowledge; it guides speaking, sleeping, and rolling in the grass. And Alzheimer's can quickly destroy the beauty of the brain and the world it interprets.

What I don't know is trapped in a convulsive time of stumbling and future loss. I look at a future of sadness and dependency. I continue to lose capability and before long this brain, racing to self-destruction, will cripple me to the point I will be unable to do the things a three-year-old does with gusto. When I can't cope, who will care for me as I slump into the shadows?

Shovel the old guy into the ashcan. Make way for the next generation. We'll need a big dumpster.

Alzheimer's is like trying to describe air. You know it is there but you cannot feel it or see it until the storm comes and the wind blows the tired, dead leaves to the ground to rot.

There were great, dusky parties in Wilmington full of loud music and chatter with friends. It was a chance for me to watch some of the people in public office with their hair down. I had always been an observer, not a dancer, a self-conscious nerd without rhythm, and tightly tuned.

During one party I got pushed on the dance floor and in a free-form manner began to dance with a woman who vibrated with sexuality. One of my friends came up and tried to push me away with a warning. Be careful of the energetic black beauty with long, smooth legs in the tight dress, he whispered.

The high school dance classes years before at Don Palini's on Washington Boulevard did not prepare me for what was in store. The woman pressed close and we danced in dizzying abandon, her knee massaging my crotch. I allowed myself to revel in the danger and the hope as she pressed herself against me. It hardened me against dancing's most basic embarrassments.

I am lonely in my dead life. Even when I am

with people and laughing with them, I am alone, isolated from the normal world, unable to remember this morning, constantly trying to recapture the moment just past. I live in a strange place of isolation, and now after years of rumination I have been cast into a place where remembering is slippery unless it happened several years ago. I feel separated from the world most of the time and I have become comfortable to sit in a room with people conversing and listen silently.

Joyce, on the other hand, has to deal with me and my slow death. She keeps her sanity by staying up late into the night with only the sound of her breathing to break the silence. She goes to bed at 4 a.m., about the same time I arise. She explains her unusual behavior as necessary to get things done. I look around and everything appears to be where it was when I last saw it. I look hard to see where the night hours have bent the world into new shapes and cleanliness. While I try to cling to the few memories left me and pine for a slow pace and simple, familiar things, Joyce is bent on creating a new world of objects to replace the one dying inside us. We have different dream worlds but we are both trying to find a place to heal.

I do not think about suicide and dying, though Alzheimer's distracts me. This is no friend, this disease, but it has taught me much about time and the world. It is difficult to create a new world without creating piles of debris.

I have grown to enjoy the surprises of everyday life and self-discovery it brings. I cling to dirt and watch marvels rise from it. I watch the robin high up in the unused greenhouse, patiently warming her five blue eggs in the fuzz of her feathers. I wait as anxiously as she to see new life. Dreams do not die even in the face of death.

There is death working away in my body. I live there in the company of fears.

Eventually Joyce, Francesco, and I came back to Virginia where I continued to write and help edit the *Delaware Spectator*, a weekly tabloid published by Ralph Morris. Every Tuesday in the early-morning darkness, Joyce drove me to Union Station in Washington and sent me off with a kiss to Wilmington where Trader or another of Ralph's assistants picked me up. The days went long into the night and when they ended, I went to Ralph's home to eat and relax. There seemed to be food available at the Morris house anytime of the day or night.

Ralph had a family so large I wondered how he and his wife, Dorina, kept track of them all. There were so many that I could barely fit in the house. I would go next door where Ralph's brother lived and sleep there.

Ralph was a great boss for a small newspaper. Not only did he have impeccable sources, he supplied encouragement when you were down. The only way I knew he was having financial troubles was when he paid me with a check and said, "Be sure to cash it before you go home." He had much sorrow, which he kept to himself, but we had a great time fighting the establishment.

Joe Brooks was one of the sterling characters Ralph found for the paper. Joe was the circulation manager. He had a glorious checkered past, which he used to hilarious account. He was a ladies' man with a wooden leg and a lover of gospel music.

Soon after I began writing "Peep's Diary," an exposé column, Joe ran into serious trouble. I had written something in "Peep's" unflattering to cops. A highly placed officer threatened Joe. He wanted to know who wrote "Peep's Diary." It was no secret but the officer reminded Joe that one more driving citation would revoke his license, leaving him with no way to get around. It was unnecessary but emblematic of the way things were done in Wilmington.

. . . .

When ability to remember is haphazard, pill-taking becomes tricky, even dangerous, as I learned the hard way.

Monday night, I made dinner, cheating as I often do, cooking prepared food. I took an Exelon tablet with the meal, as directed by my doctor. Joyce came home from work and started working in her flower garden, intending to eat later. She came in after dark and had something to eat.

When she saw I was ready for bed, she asked if I had taken my pills, as she does every night. In that short time, I forgot that I had taken the Exelon at dinner. I took another, then went upstairs and popped an Aricept into my mouth and went to bed.

Three or four hours later, around 1:30 a.m., I woke up feeling weak. Floating lights were brushing the walls of the bedroom with broken yellow patterns, an explosion of energy danced into doom.

My stomach was upset and I was disoriented. I made emotional barking sounds, dry sobs that catch in the throat, a peculiar sound I had never uttered until Alzheimer's came into my life. It is a raw language of fear, the spoken sounds of the hidden animal in the hearts of human beings. It was the only language I had in that dark room, the only way to communicate the unsettling events occurring in my fitful stomach and mind.

A vocabulary of signs and signals presented itself, vapors spiraling up through the cracks in my brain. Flying saucers in my head that no one can see, my private movies flapping in the breeze, stuck to a fence post on an open field of possibilities.

Joyce loves the night and I am an early riser, and we sometimes meet in the wee hours of the morning, but never like this. She came running when she heard my calls for help and hugged me, to give me life and comfort. When she spoke, there was fear and confusion in her voice. She was as bewildered as was I. I threw up.

I asked her where I was. I was lost and had begun to regress to another time. I called her "Mommy" and I asked where "Daddy" was in mantra-like singsong. I saw my mother where Joyce had been. I sat up in the bed and reached out to touch her in the dark air of the room but my tingling fingertips met nothing. My mother had been dead for decades, but time melted away and let me fall into a room of saints who were puffing surreal stogies.

Mommies and Daddies are familiar people to children, magical bits of flesh who work miracles. What Joyce heard in that dark night was her husband calling to his dead mother and father to give him comfort. Calling to tell them he was coming to join them.

I was well on my way to total disorientation. I threw up again.

Eventually, I thought I was in another house, a place that was completely unfamiliar. The bedroom became the place where past, present, and future met. I was in the grip of cryptic isolation.

My bowels were in torment and about to explode. Joyce helped me into the bathroom. When the cleaning of my insides ended, I was limp, unable to move. I sat on the toilet and felt my fingers and feet tingle. I looked to see if my fingertips were lit up like electrodes. I was gasping for breath.

I was too sick to stand and too uncomfortable to sit. I dropped from the toilet to the floor where I lay curled-up until the vomiting began again, dry heaves and bile. Fortunately, I had eaten so long ago hardly anything was left in my stomach. I couldn't keep myself out of the slick of bile on the floor, pumped out when I vomited, but it didn't matter; I lay in it, hardly knowing what was happening.

Gradually the disorientation subsided and my head began to clear. The radio was on in the bathroom, turned to BBC world news. I was coming back into the real world.

I was still too weak to stand, and I knew Joyce alone could not lift my 130 pounds and drag me back to the bedroom. I rolled over onto a bathmat slowly, and decided I could move myself on it by pushing off gingerly with my legs. I maneuvered the bathmat head first out of the narrow door and made a slow right turn. I rested. There was just enough strength in my legs to push my body with the bathmat under me the sixteen feet back into the bedroom, where I lifted myself up onto the bed. It was 5 a.m., three and a half hours since the ordeal began. I was exhausted. It did not take long to fall asleep.

The next day Dr. Blanchfield called it an overdose. I called it a visit to Hell.

Joyce, Francesco, and I came back to Virginia from Delaware and I got a job in journalism, several in fact, before I was tired of it and the compromises it entailed. I drove a truck for a short time for the *Washington Evening Star*. It was the most money I ever earned, over $200 a week, but I was fed up with working for other people by then and the job did not last long. I began selling plants in the fall and it produced some money. So I decided to start a nursery, selling mostly vegetable and herb plants, crops requiring little space and quick production.

In many ways, the move from Delaware signaled an end to the more reckless part of our lives, a time when we began a new life, but there was not a clear demarcation. The new life in Virginia was snuggled up to the edge of Washington, DC. It was the place both Joyce and I called home. There was no adjustment required physically, but emotionally we lost something important. It may have been slow to show itself, but we loved the people we knew in Delaware and were enchanted by the idea that human lives were worthwhile and ideas were important objects in which to believe. We recognized these things shortly after leaving, but Delaware had a way of following us and it was hard to shake the memories and the people we had loved there.

Upon returning to Virginia we were nearly penniless. We put Francesco into second grade and went to work. Joyce found a job in a department store as a shop-at-home decorator. Before the first week was history, the manager approached her. He said he had had a visit from an official who told him things to make him think she was a communist. Joyce wondered why being against an ugly, unnecessary war was subversive and why standing up for the downtrodden was wrong.

I used the money left me when my mother died to buy property in Loudoun County, Virginia, where we thought berries might grow, but quickly lost interest in those fourteen acres. Joyce and I sold the Loudoun property to a farmer who courted us for several years with annual visits and gifts of raw beef.

Eventually we settled down in the house on Ivy Street where I became content to be an urban farmer. Joyce settled into a career as an artist with a studio at the Torpedo Factory Art Center in nearby Alexandria. Francesco grew bigger and smarter and eventually left home and became a man.

Thoughts of mortality, aroused by my loss of memory, triggered the memory of a glorious time past when I hugged words and loved their feel. I resumed a life for which I once hungered and I no longer feel alone. My dream of imagination has blossomed once again.

Somewhere in the mist beyond time an immigrant baby boy from Iowa, like so many others, surprised his parents and became someone they no longer knew. The child changed in the reflected light of his time and place, and his parents were baffled by this. They remembered the boy on the sawhorse who pretended to be a cowboy, the child with arms weeping from poison ivy who needed comfort, the imaginative boy who at such an early age pretended to be a priest saying mass and used the couch as an altar. All these and other memories did not stop the child from being who he was.

They also remembered the lovely certainties of small-town life and the flat, black earth and their own childhoods, and those memories were so strong they were drawn back to the place where they started.

Memory is helpless to restore the world

the way it was, and my parents died understanding who their son had been and unsure of who he would become, and they were afraid for him. They died soon, too soon everybody said — they were only sixty when they died, four years apart, a bad heart for my father and cancer for my mother. Death is always a surprise even as it is inevitable.

Just as it was too late for the parents, so too for me now so near to my own sixty years and blighted with disease, and it is my memories now that nourish me. Back in the days when I was afraid of the dark and World War II was a fresh memory, all it took was a light and a parent's hand on my bare back to calm my fear. Now it takes more than a back rub to assuage this mental discomfort.

My father would have been ninety-one this year. I wish I could tell him I am sorry, sorry he died before his time and before we could know each other as adults. I wish I had not had to see my mother die slowly of cancer in the little hospital in Eldora, so ruined by life she could no longer suck water from a small ice cube. I am sorry it took so long to find myself and understand how much I loved them. All I have left are a few weak memories, and now it is too late for their boy.

It is frightening to lose control of your body in any way. It is especially tragic when the body's central control system, the brain, is the target of an angry destructive process that science has been unable to tame or reclaim. Memories tell us who we are and where we have been and they warm us and provide direction. In later years, the old memories remain to offer familiar anecdotes and the safety of the past.

As the brain is slowly devoured and gradually succumbs, turning the body into an empty vessel, remembering and writing are more than difficult; they are cold receptacles emptied of content. My memories are slowly disappearing from places inhabited for so long. In themselves, my memories do not compare with the great sagas of this century, the births, deaths, tumult, madness, great art and music, and the intense suffering of so many human beings. Our immortality, such as it may be, is not contained in what we dreamed or the secrets we kept; it is how our friends and loved ones remember us.

The struggle to find the words, to express myself, has become insurmountable. I must now be done with writing and lick words instead. I will soon be stripped of language and memory, existing in a shy and unsteady forbearance of nature. I am on the cusp of a new world, a place I will be unable to describe. It is the last hidden place, and marked with a headstone.

I must now wait for the silence to engulf me and take me to the place where there is no memory left and there remains no re-flexive will to live. It is lonely here waiting for memory to stop and I am afraid and tired. Hug me, Joyce, and then let me sleep.